THE INDOOR BICYCLING FITNESS PROGRAM

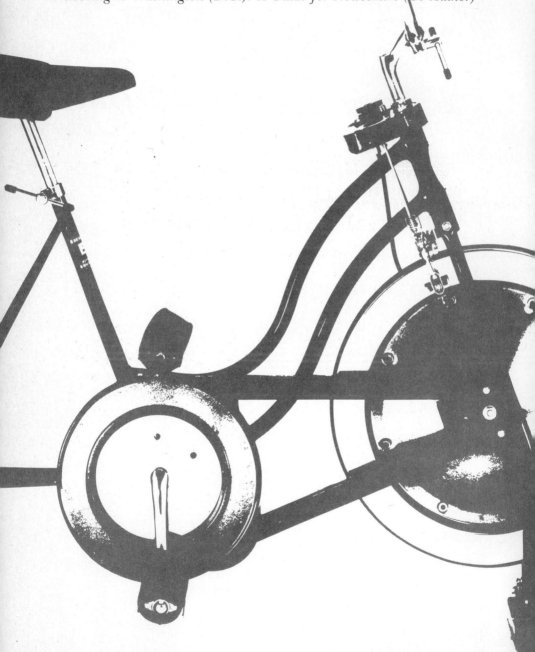

OTHER BOOKS BY JANE S. PETERS

Moving to Washington (D.C.): A Guide for Newcomers (Co-Author)

THE INDOOR BICYCLING FITNESS PROGRAM

A Complete Guide to Equipment and Exercise

Jane S. Peters

McGraw-Hill Book Company

New York St. Louis San Francisco Aukland Bogotá Guatemala
Hamburg Johannesburg Lisbon London Madrid Mexico Montreal
New Delhi Panama Paris San Juan São Paulo Singapore Sydney
Tokyo Toronto

Thanks to:

Theodore Berland for permission to reprint his skinfold chart in Chapter 7 from *The Fitness Fact Book.*

M. Evans and Company for the quote in Chapter 2 from *The Aerobics Program for Total Well-Being.* Copyright © 1982 by Dr. Kenneth H. Cooper. Reprinted by permission of the publisher, M. Evans and Company, Inc., New York, NY 10017.

Barbara George of *Velo-news* for permission to reprint the calorie chart in Chapter 7.

The Metropolitan Life Insurance Company for permission to reprint the charts in Chapter 7.

The A.M.A. for the quote in Chapter 10, reprinted with permission from *Journal of American Medical Association.*

The President's Council on Physical Fitness and Sports for permission to reprint the chart in Chapter 6.

Racer-Mate, Inc., for permission to reprint the chart in Chapter 5, and the quote in Chapter 5.

The Edison Institute's Henry Ford Museum for permission to reprint the photo of the 1886 Buffalo Home Trainer in Chapter 3.

The U.S. Weather Service for permission to reprint the heat index chart in Chapter 9.

American Health magazine for permission to reprint the quote in Appendix A.

Schwinn for portions reprinted from copyrighted materials by permission of Schwinn Bicycle Company, Chicago, Illinois, including the chart in Chapter 5.

Mazola for materials in various chapters from *Beyond Diet: Exercise Your Way to Fitness and Heart Health,* by Lenore R. Zohman, M.D., courtesy of the Mazola Nutrition/Health Information Service.

Dr. Irvin E. Faria for permission to reprint various quotes.

Dr. Ed Burke for permission to reprint various quotes.

American Youth Hostels, Inc., for permission to reprint the chart in Chapter 10.

Dr. Jack H. Wilmore for permission to reprint the chart and drawings in Chapter 7 from his book, *The Wilmore Fitness Program.*

L. Zohman, M.D., for permission to reprint the target zone chart in Chapter 5, from *Beyond Diet: Exercise Your Way to Fitness and Heart Health,* CPC International, Englewood Cliffs, New Jersey.

1 2 3 4 5 6 7 8 9   DOCDOC   8 7 6 5 4

ISBN 0-07-049589-0

Library of Congress Cataloging in Publication Data

Peters, Jane S.
  The indoor bicycling fitness program.

  Includes index.
  1. Physical fitness. 2. Cycling. 3. Cycling—
Equipment and supplies. I. Title.
GV505.P43 1985   646.7'5   84-14433
ISBN 0-07-049589-0

Book design by M.R.P. Design.

DEDICATION

To Steve Schackman. Without his support, encouragement, and, when necessary, prodding, I never would have finished this book. My second line of support was Mary Adcock, Edward Peters, and Mary Movic. Sincere thanks for their patience and positive words.

This book is also dedicated to Signe, Dorothy, Art, Dru, Jeff, and Nade Peters. Thanks also to Marie Dolan, Judy Saks, Jerry and Bea Sayper, Pat Benefield, everyone at Finan Publishing, and members of the St. Louis Writers Guild and the American Society of Journalists and Authors for their support of my writing.

Thanks to the staff at Washington University's and University City's libraries in St. Louis, and to the research staff at *Velo-news* and *Bicycling* for the many articles they photocopied for me.

Thanks also to my father (the late Dr. James A. Peters of the Smithsonian Institution) and to Dr. Bruce Fretz and Dr. Ellen Skolnick of the University of Maryland, each of whom taught me to "think like a scientist"; as well as to Dr. William J. Knaus, whose two self-help books convinced me to give this project a try.

Finally, special thanks to my sister, Jenny Peters, for an excellent preliminary editing job and astute suggestions, and to Dr. Ed Burke and McGraw-Hill's Susanne Bierds for their unwavering support. Thanks also to Elisabeth Jakab, my fine editor at McGraw-Hill.

WARNING

It is essential that the reader consult with a physician before undertaking any of the indoor bicycling fitness programs or the recommended supplementary exercises outlined in this book. Any application of the recommendations set forth in the following pages is at the reader's sole discretion and risk.

Contents

Preface

Edmund R. Burke, Ph.D.
*Technical Director, U.S. Cycling Team, United States Olympic Committee,
U.S. Cycling Federation, Inc., Colorado Springs, Colorado*
Advisor on Bicycling to the American College of Sports Medicine

The purpose of this book is to introduce you to the extraordinary world of indoor bicycling and thereby to change your life. It will show you how to become healthier and happier. It will do this no matter what shape you are currently in, and no matter how many times you may have tried—and failed—in other exercise regimens. With the proper preparation and a few precautions, you can immediately begin to change your lifestyle through an indoor bicycling program. Daily exercise is not a phenomenon that is going to disappear; its rewards are too immediate and too noticeable. Anyone who tries Jane Peters' program for a week is likely to be sold on it for life.

During this century, human beings have radically reshaped

their environment. A flood of technological advances has greatly reduced the amount of physical effort required to perform most daily activities. Although these changes have greatly benefited society, at the same time they have resulted in a deterioration in the general health and fitness levels of most people.

In the past few years, however, there has been a renewed interest in physical activity, that aspect of life so minimized by the "machine age." Many books have been published encouraging people to participate in various forms of physical activity and advising them how to do so safely and for optimum fitness.

This book will acquaint you with the information to construct an indoor bicycling fitness program tailored to your particular needs and interests. To help you achieve this, the book provides you with a working knowledge of the following:

- Aerobic fitness programs
- Potential for weight change
- The role of exercise in your lifestyle
- The psychological benefits of exercise
- How to select the best indoor bicycle for your needs
- Complete guidelines for developing an indoor bicycling fitness program
- Where to purchase your bicycle

The preparation of this book was an exciting challenge for the author. Jane Peters called upon years of experience and many miles of indoor cycling in her effort to make clear the crucial role of exercise in our daily lives. Exercise, she feels, should be considered a reward, not a punishment. Because of her considerable experience in riding and testing so many indoor bicycles, as well as exercising under many different circumstances, Ms. Peters has an expert's knowledge of the factors necessary to develop successful indoor exercise habits.

After giving the reader a comprehensive rundown of the best indoor bicycling equipment presently available, the author provides you with detailed tests and guidelines for determining your current level of physical fitness. Once you have done that, you are in a position to plan a sound personal exercise program the effectiveness of which can be evaluated by simply checking your progress as the weeks pass.

Programs for developing strength, cardiovascular fitness, flexibility, and general muscle tone are all described here in detail. Also presented are motivational tips, advice about outdoor cycling, and suggestions on how to continue your indoor program on an extended business trip or vacation.

Ms. Peters' enthusiasm is catching. Furnished with her knowledge and advice, you will soon be on your way to a more wholesome and satisfactory lifestyle. This is, quite simply, the best book on the subject of indoor bicycling to date, and will prove to be an inspiration to those readers who discover the long-term benefits of exercise in our busy society.

If cycling can be fully restored to the daily life of all Americans, it can become a vital step toward rebuilding health and vigor in all of us. . . . Let us bequeath our children more than the gadgets that surround us. The bicycle alone will not do this, but it can become a symbol of the red-blooded vigor, personal independence, and healthy mind in a healthy body that are so much needed in our beloved country today.

DR. PAUL DUDLEY WHITE, 1964

THE INDOOR BICYCLING FITNESS PROGRAM

1

Why Should You Bicycle Indoors?

Indoor bicycling has become my favorite exercise. Three years ago, I was angry with myself because I wasn't exercising regularly. It was too snowy and cold in St. Louis for outdoor bicycling; I won't run alone in the dark; and I couldn't afford dance lessons. I tried rope skipping indoors and running in place. Both aggravated my knees, and I pulled my calf muscle while running in place. Gym membership was useless, since I work an unpredictable schedule.

Accordingly, I reread everything I could find on fitness, then, with trepidation, invested in a stationary bike. Dr. Kenneth Cooper, author of the *Aerobics* books, was so unenthusiastic about indoor bicycling that I was worried. Would I be one of his anticipated dropouts?

When I started, my legs ached, and I could cycle only a few miles each day. But in a few weeks my endurance increased, and I began to accumulate miles. One day I realized that, based on my accumulated miles, I'd cycled from my St. Louis home to the Indiana border. I quickly purchased a map of the United States and began to chart my progress to Washington, D.C. (my former home).

Seven months later, I reached Washington. Next, I bicycled—indoors—across the United States. Starting from Los Angeles, I cycled to New York, a distance of 2878 miles. I then cycled—still indoors—from New York back to San Francisco. I'm now on my way around the world.

I cycle 100 to 200 miles indoors each week. Thus far, I've lost 10 pounds and more than 12 inches. I feel wonderful. My goal is to continue bicycling indoors until I'm too old to get out of bed.

Indoor bicycling is a relative newcomer to the fitness boom, but it's sweeping the United States. Almost 3 million stationary bikes are sold in this country every year, and exercise equipment sales account for more than one half of many bicycle stores' profits. Some ultramodern, sophisticated stores, in fact, sell indoor exercise equipment *only;* they don't stock outdoor bikes at all.

This book has been written for those who are contemplating a first-time investment in an indoor bike, as well as for those who already know something about them but need a useful handbook for purchasing equipment and setting up a comprehensive fitness program

This book will help you:

- Select the best indoor bicycling equipment
- Establish an exercise program to suit your particular needs
- Learn how to monitor your fitness level, while you watch it improve

Indoor bicycles are used by people in all walks of life—by movie stars to stay in shape, by the world's best athletes so that they can continue heavy workouts in bad weather, by submariners deep in the ocean's depths, and by astronauts in outer space.

Jaclyn Smith rides a Lifecycle at her local Vic Tanny's (presumably in Beverly Hills). Bernadette Peters rode an exercise bike throughout the filming of her 1983 television special.

Lon Haldeman, two-time winner of the Race Across America and holder of the men's cross-country cycling record, regularly rides an ergometer. He and his wife (Susan Notorangelo, holder of the women's cross-country record and women's record holder for the 750-mile Paris/Brest/Paris race) alternate use of that bike. Lon has also trained for many thousands of hours on rollers.

Lynn Adams and Kathy McMullen of the Ladies Professional Golf Association take collapsible exercise bikes when they travel around the country, to ensure a guaranteed, predictable workout wherever they are. Tennis pro Arthur Ashe also puts in the miles on an indoor bike.

Members of numerous sports teams, including the Detroit Tigers, Philadelphia Flyers, and Chicago Bears, ride ergometers. Many players on the St. Louis Cardinals baseball team, including coach Whitey Herzog, ride exercise bikes as part of their training. So do the Los Angeles Dodgers and New York Yankees.

Even crew members on a Polaris submarine have cycled "indoors": in one fitness study conducted by the U.S. Navy, two exercise bikes were placed between a couple of missile tubes—the only available space on board the sub.

The indoor bicycle has actually gone into outer space. Restraint systems have been developed for bicycle ergometers so that astronauts can use them under zero-gravity conditions or in a position that's not upright. Two people, in fact, literally rode indoor bikes around the world. NASA astronaut Alan Bean rode an exercise bike during *Skylab II*'s 1973 flight—an 80-minute orbit around the earth. Charles Conrad did the same on an earlier flight that lasted 110 minutes.

Why has such an illustrious crowd adapted indoor cycling? And why should you join them? Because indoor bicycling requires little time, keeps your muscles toned, helps you lose weight and keep it off, is easily done at home any time, and provides outstanding aerobic exercise.

It's a simple, easy, satisfying, enjoyable, and rewarding form of exercise. In fact, indoor cycling may be the most convenient, easily accessible exercise ever invented. You don't have to leave home, don't even need to step outside your front door, to exercise.

You can ride your bike at 6:30 A.M., before showering for work; at midnight, before you climb into bed; in the afternoon, before your children get home from school; just before lunch or dinner to curb your appetite; or at 9:00 P.M. while you read your favorite suspense novel.

You'll never have to wait in line at the gym, walk home after you've finished your laps, or exit, sweaty and smelly, from aerobic dancing in a church basement that lacks a shower.

Indoor cycling can provide you with a comprehensive exercise program that can be adapted to virtually any schedule and any circumstance.

Additionally, when you bike indoors, you won't waste time gathering and locating exercise equipment. You won't need to search for racquets, balls, or bats, check your 10-speed bike's gears and brakes, or dry out a clammy bathing suit.

No matter where you live, you can follow an indoor bicycling program. Even if you should relocate numerous times, your indoor bike will accompany you. You can live in the Arctic wilderness, and bike; in the Amazon jungles, and bike; in a high-rise condo in New York City, and bike; or in the middle of an Illinois cornfield, and bike.

You won't have to worry about choosing a new home that's near a gym, health club, jogging trail, or swimming pool. Since your indoor bicycling program is self-contained, you won't ever again have to rely on outside facilities to maintain your fitness level.

And you can follow your exercise program no matter what the weather. You won't be affected by pouring rain, 6 inches of snow, 99°F and 100 percent humidity, a pollution alert, or even a tornado watch. You'll just pedal away on your indoor bike, oblivious to it all.

Cycling indoors is also one of the safest exercises that exists. The probability of being injured on, or falling off, an indoor bike is extremely low. Even if such an unusual event occurs, you're at home and in virtually no danger.

You also won't experience the jarring or pounding sensations constantly felt by runners. Shin splints, runner's knee, water in the ears from too much swimming, tennis elbow, and similar sports injuries are impossible with an indoor bicycling program.

Indoor bicycling also offers none of the hazards of outdoor cycling. You won't dodge or avoid traffic, fight off dogs nipping at your ankles, have to avoid bumpy potholes or watch out for motorists who might toss sticks or beer cans at you, or groan when you approach huge hills. And you'll never be involved in a serious collision, as you might be on a 10-speed bike.

Then too, cycling indoors can be easily stopped if problems arise. Have you, for example, ever begun a 10-mile run, pulled a muscle after 5 miles, and limped home? Or did you try a 50-mile bicycle tour when you weren't yet in condition for such a trip, then flagged a passing truck to get home? If so, the advantages of cycling indoors are obvious. On an indoor bike you finish *exactly* where you started. If you feel exhausted, just dismount and rest.

Indoor bicycling is relatively inexpensive, too. The total cost is less than most racquet sports, golf, dancing, or swimming. And remember, when your entire family rides an indoor bike, the cost per person is minimal. The cost of the initial equipment covers your family's exercise needs. With other sports, however, expenses double or triple when the entire family participates.

Should you add accessories to your indoor bike (such as a reading stand, downturned handlebars, or racing seat), your investment is still low. Only a few accessories are necessary—although some of the unnecessary ones are a lot of fun.

You also won't have to corral a partner or organize a team, and you'll never pay court fees or fees for lessons. Just mount your bike and start pedaling.

Only a small amount of space is needed for a stationary bike or ergometer (approximately 2 feet by 5 feet). If you should decide to purchase rollers or a wind-load simulator, you'll need slightly more space, approximately 2 feet by 6 feet (about the size of your 10-speed bike).

But you may not need to purchase an indoor bike. Nowadays, indoor bikes are available practically everywhere. Using the fitness programs set up in this book, you can exercise on any available equipment. Health clubs provide bikes for members, as do YMCAs, and indoor biking is in vogue at health spas and resorts. Many hotels and motels offer exercise bikes to guests, and at some you're allowed to ride in the privacy of your room.

Indoor bicycling is an especially enjoyable form of exercise when you're traveling, since you'll never have to jog through dangerous, unfamiliar neighborhoods, search for a gym offering daily rates, find a swimming pool where you can swim laps, or locate a dance class that fits your schedule.

You might even, as many Americans have, use an indoor bike at work. Your company might have purchased one for the office or for the gym or exercise room. Ergometers, for example, can be found at the General Electric Employee Fitness Center, ITT Employee Fitness Center, and the Levi-Strauss Employee Fitness Center.

Indoor bicycling is one of the few fitness programs you'll never grow too old to enjoy. In fact, there's virtually no reason ever to discontinue your indoor cycling. There are, however, many reasons that encourage you to *continue* cycling as you age. Your bones will remain strong and your muscles supple, which helps prevent osteoporosis, a bone disease that often plagues senior citizens. If your hearing worsens or your vision deteriorates with age, you can still bicycle indoors. Many deaf and blind people regularly ride indoor bikes.

You may also be interested to learn that indoor bicycling is used for rehabilitation. Doctors frequently prescribe indoor biking for people recovering from heart attacks or strokes, who need exercise yet can't participate in most outdoor activities. An indoor bicycling program is often prescribed for people recovering from knee, hip, and ankle operations. Few other types of exercises can be employed for this purpose, since people's joints often cannot bear any weight after such operations. (See Chapter 10 for more information.)

Bicycling indoors also develops physical skills that can easily be transferred outdoors. "I don't want to bicycle indoors all year," says one indoor cyclist. "I adore the crisp spring and fall air. I want to cycle outside then, exploring country roads, enjoying the fine weather." Happily, the stamina you develop from indoor bike workouts helps you explore the outdoors. You'll probably outdistance your friends who didn't ride their bikes all winter, and your leg, heart, arm, and other muscles will be in terrific shape.

You'll never regret your choice of indoor bicycling as a long-term fitness program. And when you choose to cycle indoors, you'll join millions of other people—here in the United States and throughout the world—who maintain their physical health and mental well-being with the best form of exercise ever created.

2

Why Indoor Bicycling's Good for Your Body and Your Mind

Exercise physiologists and psychologists have for many years used bicycle ergometers to measure the benefits accumulating from other kinds of exercise. However, it's only recently that researchers have turned their attention to the benefits of indoor bicycling itself.

Research related to indoor cycling has also been conducted by physiologists interested in cycling as an amateur or professional sport. Some of the most interesting studies, in fact, have been done on Olympic and world-class cyclists, and many of these studies also apply to us slower folk.

Studies on supercyclists (as well as on average human beings) commonly are conducted on three kinds of machines: (1) bicycle ergometers, precisely calibrated stationary bikes that measure the work you're doing with scientific accuracy; (2) wind-load simulators, squirrel-cage-type gadgets that attach to the back wheel of your 10-speed bike to provide resistance, a breezy effect, and a precise measurement of workload; or (3) scientifically calibrated rollers (a contraption consisting primarily of three drums on which you balance your 10-speed bike while you ride).

The latest development in the analysis of the physiology of bicycling is, naturally, the computer. Dr. Peter Cavanagh, of the Applied Research Laboratory at Pennsylvania State University, has a computer that can receive 2200 pieces of information per minute about a cyclist's performance. Once a complete analysis of various tests is obtained, a researcher has about 400,000 pieces of information!

At this lab, you pedal with a computer screen set up in front of you and you receive immediate feedback as to what you're doing wrong (or right). Not surprisingly, with such expensive equipment, the primary users are members of the U.S. National Cycling Team and of racing clubs.

Indoor bicycling is basically an aerobic exercise; the proven positive changes that result from such exercise include:

- Better sleep
- Stronger joints
- Increased energy and stamina
- Stronger, more supple muscles
- Stronger bones (from the action of strong muscles)
- Higher output from your heart, with less rise in pulse
- A lowered resting pulse
- Improved circulation
- Growth of new blood vessels and capillaries
- Increased oxygen-carrying capacity of your blood
- Better digestion
- Reduced constipation
- Control or reduction of weight, and avoidance of winter weight gain
- Reduced levels of unhealthy cholesterol
- Deeper breathing while you exercise
- Better heat acclimatization (when you exercise in the heat, rather than in air conditioning)

• Stronger back muscles (especially if you use dropped handlebars on your indoor bike)

• Reduced accumulation of painful lactic acid in your muscles, even when you exercise at the same intensity

• Reduced triglyceride levels

• Faster recovery after exercise of both your heart and blood pressure

• Lower oxygen consumption for a given amount of work, and a greater maximum oxygen consumption (a measure of your lungs' capacity to take in oxygen and give off carbon dioxide)

• For women, easier pregnancies

Most researchers agree that at least six weeks of *aerobic* training, at a frequency of at least three times a week, are necessary before these beneficial changes begin to occur. The word "aerobic" means "with oxygen," and it applies to any continuous exercise that makes your heart beat faster while you breathe more deeply. To qualify as aerobic, exercise must be continued longer than a few minutes. Thus, your pulse may increase and you may puff a little when you lift weights, but you're not performing aerobic work.

Aerobic exercises include continuous bicycling, running, swimming, walking, and cross-country skiing, among others. Indoor bicycling, however, is the most easily measured (and monitored) of these exercises. Glenn Goldfinger, of New York Unversity's Medical Center Institute of Rehabilitative Medicine, claims that indoor bicycling is the most perfect way to develop an aerobic exercise program.

However, research studies also indicate that your fitness improves most rapidly if you can combine aerobic and *anaerobic* exercise. "Anaerobic" exercise is short-term, *very* intense work that is carried out, *without oxygen,* to the limits of your endurance. You can continue it for only a short period, since when your muscles run out of oxygen, lactic acid accumulation causes your muscle cells to become so acidic that they fatigue almost immediately, and the pain forces you to stop. It *is* possible to cycle both aerobically and anaerobically. While the fitness programs recommended in Chapter 5 are primarily aerobic, supplementary anaerobic programs are included as well. However, the main emphasis in any fitness program must remain on aerobic exercise.

Numerous studies substantiate the benefits of aerobic exercise. Some are mentioned here, others throughout this book. For example, a 24-year study of 17,000 male Harvard graduates, recently reported in the *Journal of the American Medical Association,* emphasizes the importance of engaging in regular aerobic exercise—even if it's just a fast walk every other day. The researchers found that regular exercise helps prevent heart and lung disease and prolongs life. A similar study of 6000 men and women, conducted by the Dallas Institute for Aerobics Research, found that physically fit people were less likely to suffer from hypertension.

Another study, reported in *Metabolism,* found that young women who followed a 10-week bicycle ergometer training program consisting of 30 minutes per session three times per week increased the ability of their lungs to process oxygen and carbon dioxide, as well as their capacity for exercise. The women's percentage of body fat was determined by underwater weighing, then remeasured after the 10-week program ended. Significant reductions in body fat were found, and their resting heart rates also went down significantly.

Other research has shown that aerobic exercise improves your ability to tolerate heavy workloads, increases your lung capacity, reduces your stress level, and promotes relaxation and better sleep.[1]

Research also indicates that people who regularly engage in aerobic exercise don't come down with infections as often as do nonexercisers. It's suspected that part of the reason may be what's

---

[1] A study reported in *Clinical Cardiology* found that a five-week fitness training regimen significantly increased maximal work tolerance and reduced the subjects' heart rate both at rest and during exercise.

Another study, reported by the National Technical Information Service, used an exercise program combining bicycle ergometer workouts and running. The subjects, normal men aged 25 to 35, showed definite increases in their work capacity: lung capacity increased, heart rate slowed, maximum oxygen consumption increased by 14 percent, and stress levels decreased.

Research conducted at the University of California indicated that bicycling, walking, and jogging (all of which are sustained, rhythmic aerobic exercises) promote relaxation and better sleep. Another study reported in *Psychophysiology* found that male volunteers who went without sleep for a period of time recovered better if they bicycled. The exercisers were able to spend more total time in sleep (while recovering from a sleep deficit) than were the nonexercisers.

known as *endogenous pyrogen,* a protein that increases body temperature and creates an environment hostile to bacteria. Thus, regular aerobic exercise can cause a rise in your body's temperature that could aid your resistance to infection for hours after a workout.

Another study found that as physical fitness increases, fewer white blood cells must be mobilized before the body's immune response is activated. When fitness is low, however, more white blood cells are needed for the body to produce its immune response. The findings also indicate that for healthy people, better fitness levels compensate for the effects of stress.

Psychologists and psychiatrists examining the effects of indoor cycling on mental health have found an impressive amount of evidence indicating that regular aerobic exercise can produce improved mental acuity; enhanced stress tolerance and reduced tension; less depression; better ability to concentrate; increased self-confidence; less anxiety and irritability; a more positive attitude toward your body; better mental alertness; and greater emotional stability.

In short, you'll feel good in *many* ways mentally when you engage in a regular indoor bicycling program. Many people, in fact, become friendlier and more gregarious as they continue their fitness program. Obviously, it's not simply your muscles and heart that benefit from regular aerobic exercise; it's also your mind, emotions, and stress level.

In his recent book *The Aerobics Program for Total Well-Being,* Dr. Kenneth Cooper cites research conducted by Florida psychiatrist Dr. Ray Killinger. Killinger's work indicates that "in conjunction with exercise, greater originality of thought is shown, the duration of concentration increases, and the mental response time is quicker. Also the person who is aerobically fit has the ability to change subject material quickly and more effectively than an unconditioned person. A fit individual can carry more ideas simultaneously and has greater mental tenacity when trying to resolve tough and prolonged questions."[2]

---

[2]Dr. Cooper's review of the literature in the *Annals of Clinical Research* concluded that improved physical fitness led to less depression, less hypochondria, a more positive attitude toward life, and improved self-image.

A study conducted at England's University of Keele followed male coronary patients

Recently, researchers have focused on the effects on mental health of certain hormones released during exercise. The latest research is on *endorphins*, hormones thought to cause the "high" that people who exercise aerobically often experience. Endorphin levels can increase as high as five times above normal during strenuous exercise, and these hormonal levels may remain elevated for hours *after* exercise.

"Our soul is in our brain," said bicyclist Dr. Paul Dudley White, "a fact to which our clergy and psychiatrists should pay more attention. Our brain is nourished by our heart and our active muscles. Bicycles are an answer for both brain and body. If more of us rode them, we would have a sharp reduction in the use of tranquilizers and sleeping pills."

---

with an average age of approximately 50. Patients who exercised on a bicycle ergometer showed higher morale than that of patients who didn't exercise at all. In addition, the exercisers' anxiety scores fell more than did those of the nonexercisers. One of the most important effects of exercise on these patients was increased self-confidence.

One study at New Mexico State University found that young men who engaged in a weight-training program had a significant improvement in five out of nine measures of self-concept. How objectively *successful* the men were in their weight training did not significantly affect the extent of their personality change.

A study by Dr. Robert Conroy found that a six-week fitness program produced reduced depression and increased the sense of accomplishment of psychiatric patients.

Anxiety can be reduced by bicycle ergometer exercise. One study found that female college students who watched a disturbing movie on industrial accidents were less anxious when they exercised on a bicycle while watching than were women who sat still.

3

Indoor Bicycling Equipment

BACKGROUND

If you think all indoor bicycles resemble those flimsy, fragile, bouncing ones that you've seen in your local discount or department store, you're wrong. High-quality equipment for indoor cycling has burgeoned in the last few years. Today, you can choose between a stationary bicycle, a bicycle ergometer, a wind-load simulator, and rollers.

A huge industry also caters to the cyclist's insatiable desire for accessories. You can improve your indoor cycling program by purchasing handlebar and seat padding, special clothing, reading stands, and even complex computers that will calculate your every move.

To produce an adequate aerobic effect, your indoor cycling equipment must have the following features:

- A strong, stable, well-made design
- A method to increase and reduce the tension level, usually a dial
- A speedometer or tachometer [tachometers measure the revolutions per minute (rpm) of your feet]
- An odometer, to keep track of your mileage
- A timer
- An easy-to-use control panel

If you purchase cycling equipment without these features, you're more likely to give up on your exercise program.

Research studies on "perceived exertion" explain why you need to have a reliable tension control dial on your indoor bike. Basically, such studies conclude that just because you *perceive* a particular workout to be more difficult than the one you did yesterday doesn't mean that it *is*. Your perception may be affected by how little you had to eat for breakfast, how much alcohol you drank last night, or how tired your muscles are from yesterday's exercise. In other words, you can't adequately "feel" how much work you're doing, nor can you judge the difficulty of a particular workout by how it "feels."

Please don't rush out to your local discount store and buy a flimsy bike. Don't waste money on those silly exercisers you see in mail-order catalogs, the ones where you lie on the floor and pedal a thin metal piece with your feet. Ignore the many ads for foldaway bicycles that are nothing more than two pieces of wood (or metal) with a hinge.

Even if you have a tiny apartment, you can find space for a normal-sized exercise bike or ergometer. Those cheap imitations are just that—cheap. Rich Morris, owner of St. Louis's Maplewood Bicycle shop, says: "Buying a cheap bike is a total waste of money. You might as well take a walk and save the money." He continues, "There's so much junk out there that we refuse to repair certain brands since they're so poorly made."

The high-quality indoor exercise equipment I recommend in this book will ensure that your indoor bicycling closely simulates the "outdoor riding" experience. If, for example, your legs should be in the wrong position, you'll use muscles that don't match those used on a 10-speed bike and your cycling will be more physiologically inefficient than necessary. You'll waste energy, and your feet will wander all over, if you don't replace the common plastic pedals with the metal "rattrap" kind (the ones with holes), toe clips (metal contraptions that fit over your toes and hold them in the scientifically determined best location), and leather straps that keep your feet securely in the clips. Without clips, you also won't use the large muscles in the back of your legs as efficiently. You should also have downturned handlebars and a narrow "racing" seat. If you ride an indoor bike with upturned handlebars and a wide seat, your arms, elbows, and shoulders will never gain the strength you need for everyday life—or even for riding on the road, should you eventually decide to do so.

Naturally, price must be a consideration when choosing indoor cycling equipment. The bikes included here are priced from $250 to $600, although I've included a brief section about others that retail for more.

In my opinion, the equipment listed in this book is the best available today. For the fitness programs detailed here, bikes that are triple action (models that resemble horseback riding) or electrically powered are not suitable, and under no circumstances should you purchase equipment that comes without a guarantee. Since I mention at least two or three models in every major category of indoor bicycling equipment, however, you'll have plenty of choice.

I strongly recommend that you purchase your equipment at a reputable local bicycle store. They'll assemble it, check the instrumentation, and stand behind their equipment. Many bike shops rent indoor bikes on a lease/purchase plan, so you can try out a bike for a month or so before you buy. And virtually every shop will give you a trial ride on their equipment so that you can test the feel.

If you decide to purchase items by mail order, choose a high-quality catalog company that specializes in bicycling equipment (see Appendix F), or buy directly from the manufacturer, who will stand behind the product. Don't make your purchase at a discount store, department store, or five-and-dime. The staff knows little about fitness or bicycling, and they can't fix your equipment if it breaks down.

Keep in mind that you may want to upgrade your equipment

as your fitness increases. If you should purchase a stationary bike, you might find, as I did, that after a year or two you want to move up to an ergometer, which measures your improved fitness *precisely*. At that time, you might also think about a set of rollers, since they'll improve your outdoor riding skills and increase your confidence in dealing with problems on the road.

You might also find that a wind-load simulator (WLS) appeals to you if you've purchased a 10-speed bike and occasionally cycle outdoors. The resistance and "windy" feel of a WLS almost convinces you that you're outside, even if you're riding in your basement while winter winds howl outdoors. So don't presume that the indoor bicycling equipment you purchase to begin your program will be the *last* piece you ever buy. It might be—but it might *not* be, either. In fact, many of the top U.S. bicycle racers train at home using a variety of different devices, each for different reasons.

Compare the pros and cons of various types of indoor bicycling equipment, read the next sections on choosing the various types of equipment, then take a trial ride at your local bicycle shop. You'll soon be ready to begin your fitness program.

PROS AND CONS OF DIFFERENT EQUIPMENT

Stationary Bicycles

A stationary bike is similar to what you'd get if you took a 10-speed bike, removed the backwheel, placed it on sturdy crossbar legs, then added a tension device, chain cover, speedometer, odometer, and sometimes, a timer. The ones I recommend feature a heavy flywheel which stabilizes the bike and produces a feeling similar to riding outdoors.

Pros

Inexpensive.

Don't have to own a 10-speed bike.

Takes up little space.

Easily moved.

No calibration checks necessary.

Good for starting an indoor cycling fitness program.

Available at hotels, on ships, at health spas, and so on, as you travel.

You can read while you're riding.

Easily adjusted for all family members.

Cons

No way to measure your fitness level precisely; you must rely on your pulse.

Exact workload cannot be repeated the next day (as it can be on an ergometer).

No fan included.

Many cycling accessories don't work on them, since there are no bicycle spokes.

Distance and angle of handlebars and seat may not simulate riding outdoors.

Bicycle Ergometers

Often the only thing that distinguishes an ergometer from a stationary bicycle is the device that measures your workload. An ergometer features a scientifically accurate, precisely calibrated workload measuring device that lets you calculate exactly how hard you're working and precisely how many calories you're using, and lets you duplicate the same workload tomorrow. This device adds to the ergometer's cost, naturally, but you may find, as I have, that accuracy is worth the extra cost.

Pros

Instruments allow precise measurement of fitness levels.

You can repeat the exact workload tomorrow, since the measurements are scientifically accurate.

You don't have to own a 10-speed bike.

Available at hotels, on ships, at health spas, and so on, as you travel.

You can read while you're riding.

You can accurately calculate the calories you've used.

You can test your fitness regularly and compare it with standards for your age, since you have precise workload measurements (some ergometers have booklets that explain how to do this).

You can compare your rate of exercise with other activities such as jogging or running (see Table 5–4).

Easily adjusted for all family members.

Cons

Expensive to extremely expensive.

You may have to recalibrate it periodically, or you may have to take it to a bike shop for calibration.

Some measure workload accurately only at certain rpm levels (which is a problem if you prefer to cycle faster or slower).

No fan included (except on Schwinn's Air-Dyne).

Many cycling accessories don't work on them, since there are no bicycle spokes.

Distance and angle of handlebars and seat may not simulate outdoor cycling.

Wind-Load Simulators

To use a wind-load simulator, you take off your 10-speed bike's front wheel. Then you clamp the bike into an odd-looking contraption that securely holds the bike's front fork and rear frame. A bar supports the bike's weight, while crossbars provide stability. A wind-load simulator typically has a small roller on which your bike's rear wheel turns, and a couple of round squirrel-cage attachments that ride on either side of the back wheel to provide a form of resistance or tension control.

Pros

Inexpensive.

Built-in cooling fan effect.

Has instruments that allow precise measurement of fitness.

You can repeat the exact workload tomorrow, since the measurements are scientifically accurate.

No balancing skills needed (as they are on rollers).

Uses your own 10-speed bike.

Gives the feeling of outdoor cycling by the wind-resistance squirrel cages.

You can read while you're riding.

You can accurately calculate the calories you've used (see Figure 5–2).

Can be used as a bike repair stand.

Cons

You must own a 10-speed bike.

If you're traveling, you must bring both the WLS and your bike.

Noisy.

You must reattach all equipment you've taken off your bike (including the front wheel) if you want to ride outdoors.

If other family members want to use the WLS, you must take your bike off and put theirs on.

Might not fit unusual bikes (15-speeds, tandems, etc.).

Rollers

Rollers usually consist of three cylindrical drums that can be spaced to fit your 10-speed bike's dimensions. The drums are supported by a frame and connected with belts to ensure that the front drum revolves simultaneously with the back ones. You ride rollers by balancing your bike's front wheel on the front drum while you balance your rear wheel on the back drums.

Pros

Inexpensive.

Uses your own 10-speed bike.

Teaches excellent balance.

Provides an instant check on your bike's mechanical condition.

Teaches you to ride a perfectly straight line.

Teaches a much smoother ride, since you must ride smoothly to stay on the rollers.

Teaches you to change gears without weaving, and to control the bike while you're changing gears.

Can be used to check miscellaneous adjustments on your bike instead of your having to do it out on the road (i.e., seat, handlebars, gears, brakes, etc.).

Teaches you to reduce any tendency to pedal more with one leg than the other, since it shows up in your ability to balance.

Cons

No way to measure your fitness level precisely; you must rely on heart rate.

Most models don't have resistance attachments.

You must own a 10-speed bike.

Your bike must be in virtually perfect condition; if it's not, you probably won't be able to stay on the rollers.

Your tires must always be highly inflated (if they're not, it's very difficult to pedal), and so you'll probably have to purchase a heavy-duty pump.

Your wheels must be almost exactly round.

Needs quite a bit of space to avoid injury.

Difficult to read while riding.

Your balancing skills must be excellent.

Can be quite difficult to learn to ride (especially if you're not a cyclist or are a senior citizen).

Noisy.

If you're traveling, you must bring both the rollers and your bike.

No fans (except on Kreitler rollers).

Roller belt could break while you're cycling.

Flat tire could throw you off the rollers.

Probably the most boring indoor cycling equipment.

Roller-riders sweat more profusely than other indoor cyclists.

You must reattach all equipment that you've taken off your bike when you ride outdoors.

Roller-riding is like "bicycling on ice" to some people.

Tires wear out more quickly than on the road.

Rollers might not roll if you have thick carpeting.

EQUIPMENT

Stationary Bicycles

Bicycles have been ridden as indoor exercise devices practically since their invention. On a recent visit to Detroit's marvelous Henry Ford Museum, I came upon the 1886 "Buffalo Home Trainer" in their fascinating bicycle display. The Buffalo, an exercise bike which resembles a unicycle (see Figure 3–1), must have been even more difficult to ride than today's rollers!

Stationary bikes and ergometers were mentioned in the medical literature by 1912. Those research-oriented bikes were de-

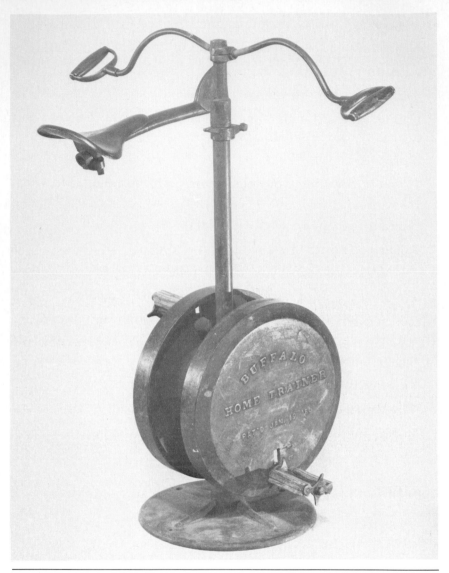

Figure 3–1   The 1886 Buffalo Home Trainer, the first known exercise bike. *(Courtesy of Henry Ford Museum, The Edison Institute, Dearborn, MI.)*

signed with a racing seat, flywheel, rubber pedals, and a stable wooden or metal base. They actually weren't too different from those recommended in this chapter.

Over the years, indoor bicycles have also been used as a power source in the United States and, more recently, in less developed countries. An "ordinary" high-wheel bicycle was set up to power a sewing machine at the turn of the century, and handsaws and grinding wheels have been powered by indoor bicycle contraptions. Past uses of indoor bicycling equipment were limited only by the owner's imagination and by the work that needed to be done.

Stationary bikes are far more sophisticated today, yet the basic principle remains the same. One wheel of an outdoor bike is removed, a secure base is added, and a brake system or cloth belt is added for resistance, as are a speedometer, odometer, and timer.

Test riding your new bike before you purchase it is essential. Even though the ratings in this book are thorough, nothing substitutes for the feel of a bike when you test it. I especially recommend testing if you're either very tall or very short, or have extremely long or short legs or arms.

Consider the noise level of the bike you have in mind. Some bikes are so noisy that you'd probably be evicted from your apartment the first time you rode one, whereas others are so quiet that you barely hear them across the room.

Where you plan to place the bike in your apartment will affect your concern about noise. My indoor bike is in my bedroom, a sun porch located over a downstairs entryway, so any noise would bother my neighbors only when they're standing in the hall. In another apartment, I placed my bike at the end of a long hallway, on a landing that headed upstairs (St. Louis has *huge* apartments). Again, my neighbors heard cycling noises only when they walked to the end of their hall. So far, I've had no complaints.

Besides noise levels, you should compare each stationary bike on the following variables, all of which are extremely important to your long-term enjoyment:

- Length of warranty.
- Price.
- Whether the bike has a timer, odometer, and speedometer, and whether they are resettable. (Note whether they measure in kilometers or miles.)
- Overall construction quality.

- Heaviness and balance of flywheel.
- Overall stability, with no bouncing, jerking, or flexing of frame or posts.
- Handlebars, seat, and pedals that can easily be replaced or that come in racing style. (For a detailed explanation, see Chapter 4.)
- Quality of the tension control system. If you make small adjustments on the tension knob, do you produce equally small tension increases? If not, you'll either find yourself working harder or easier than you want.
- Ease of assembly, especially if the bike won't be assembled at your bike store.
- Total weight.
- Whether the bike has solid, leveling feet.
- Whether a tachometer is included, and what type it is.
- Convenience of the control box.
- Whether you get an outdoors feeling as you ride.
- The bike's portability.
- Where you'll go for repairs.
- Any helpful extras.

If you're debating between two models, rent each one for a month or so. An at-home trial can help you clarify your likes and dislikes better than a store trial. Most bicycle shops and fitness equipment dealers rent indoor bikes, and often they'll deduct your first few month's rent from the purchase price. Industry statistics show that virtually everyone who rents an indoor bike ends up buying it.

Remember that your stationary bike will quite possibly be a lifetime investment. Buy a good one. If you're concerned about the price, remember that in the long run your indoor bike will be cheaper than a 10-speed bike. Owners of 10-speed bikes constantly replace brakes, spokes, tires, and wheels, and often add panniers, water bottles, and tool bags. Then, too, you'll never replace anything on a stationary bike due to a collision, since you'll never have an accident.

If you're still bothered about the price of a stationary bike, consider splitting the cost with a neighbor. Keep the bike in one person's garage, and schedule times when each of you will use it.

However, before you rush out to purchase a stationary bike, I'd suggest that you read the section on bicycle ergometers. Some of the least expensive ergometers cost about the same as the best stationary bikes, and you might decide that their ability to measure your exercise workload and calorie consumption precisely justify the additional cost.

The stationary bikes listed here are arranged alphabetically by manufacturer's name. All are of approximately equal quality— read each description for individual variations.

Monark/Universal Fitness Exercise Cycle 867 ($450). This sturdy, well-made, tubular steel Swedish bike, shown in Figure 3–2, weighs 60 pounds and has a one-year warranty on parts from Universal Fitness.

The speedometer measures up to 60 kilometers per hour, but there's no tachometer or timer. The cumulative odometer also measures in kilometers.

The 867's flywheel is heavy, made of 60 pounds of solid aluminum. Tension is controlled by a tough nylon strap around the flywheel. You adjust the workload using a calibrated dial that's numbered from 0 to 6. On this bike, you can reproduce your workload of the previous day (i.e., if you used a setting of 2 yesterday, you could work at 2 again today), but there's no objective measure of *how much* that load is as there would be on an ergometer.

Handlebars adjust up and down, and are dropped and comfortable. You can raise their height from 39 inches to 42.5 inches. Optional bars that look like those on the Mark II (see the upcoming section on ergometers) are available. The handlebars and seat are quick-release.

This Monark comes with a racing saddle, and the calibrated seat post can be adjusted at 1-inch intervals. The total post length is 435 millimeters.

Now available for this model is an "infinite tension control" device. The manufacturer says that it "completely eliminates any sudden, sharp changes in resistance by providing a full range of tension adjustments."

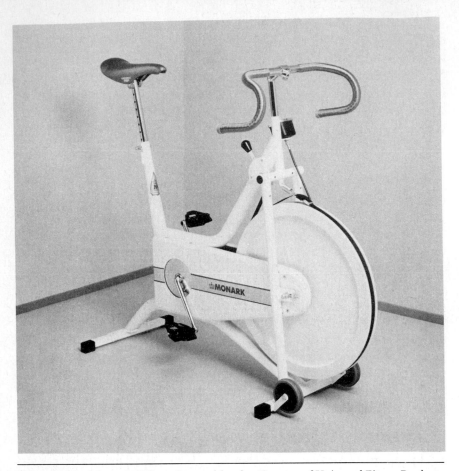

Figure 3–2 Monark 867 stationary bicycle. *(Courtesy of Universal Fitness Products, Plainview, NY.)*

The 867's ball-bearing pedals are made of plastic without toe clips or straps. They can be replaced, if you wish.

Although this is a solid, heavy bike, it can be moved around on two small front wheels and the flywheel. The body is the same as that for the more expensive 868 ergometer.

Universal Fitness has a toll-free number for repairs (800–645–7554). They have dealers in some states who do repairs, or you can buy spare parts and do it yourself (most indoor bikes are not that complicated), or you can ship the bike back to them.

Basically identical to the 868 ergometer (all that's missing is the workload monitor—see the section on ergometers), the 867 is an excellent, quiet bike.

Monark/Universal Fitness Home Cycle 875 ($330). This well-made Swedish stationary bike weighs 55 pounds (see Figure 3–3). Universal Fitness offers a one-year warranty on parts for this tubular steel bike. The speedometer measures in kilometers, as does the odometer. There's no tachometer or timer.

It's a quiet bike, typical of Monarks. No leveling feet are available on this bike.

The small, 40-pound flywheel is made of solid aluminum. Tension control comes from a nylon strap around the flywheel that's controlled from a dial; the chain is protected, and pedals are plastic, without toe clips or straps. The pedals can be replaced, if you wish.

Foam-covered handlebars are adjustable to virtually any position (a new feature). Both handlebars and seat are quick-release. The oversized, soft seat can be replaced with a racing saddle, and the post is adjustable at 1-inch intervals. The total post length is 435 millimeters.

Universal has a toll-free number for repairs (800-645-7554). They have dealers in some states who do repairs, or you can buy spare parts and do it yourself (most indoor bikes are not that complicated), or you can ship the bike back to them.

The low frame design makes for especially easy mounting. You can roll this bike around on its front wheels.

Overall, a well-made, sturdy little bike.

Schwinn/Excelsior XR-7 ($250). All Schwinn bikes come with a lifetime guarantee and a free 30-day checkup. The XR-7, shown in Figure 3–4, is the least expensive bike rated. It weighs 55 pounds and has a medium noise level (which is less on the 1984 model—see below). Its base is extremely stable, and it has leveling feet, a nice feature that's lacking on most indoor bikes.

The speedometer records in miles, but there's no tachometer. The timer can be set up to 30 minutes, and a bell sounds when you're finished. The odometer records miles, but cannot be reset.

The XR-7's flywheel is an all-metal inertia type and is heavy. Handlebars are quick-release, adjust up and down, and are easily

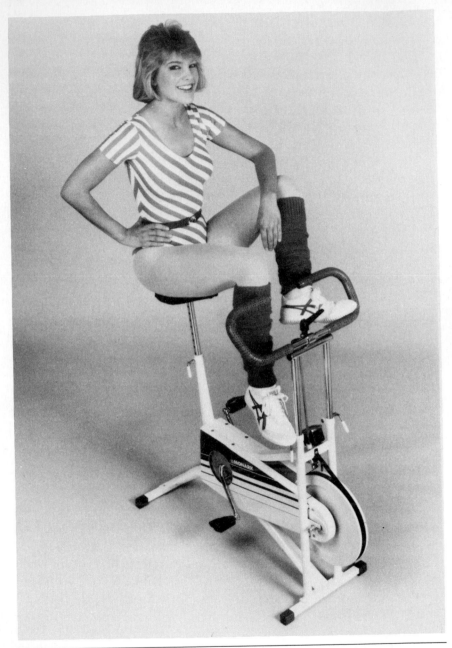

Figure 3–3   Monark 875 stationary bicycle. *(Courtesy of Universal Fitness Products, Plainview, NY.)*

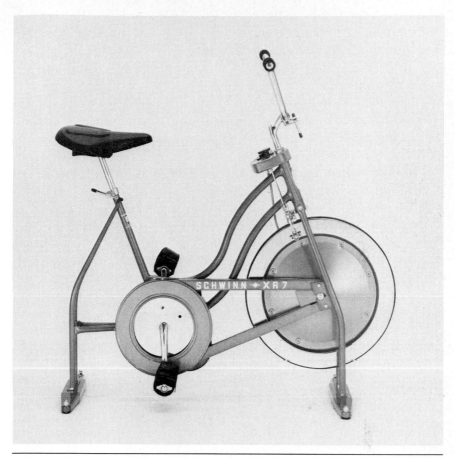

Figure 3–4 Schwinn/Excelsior XR-7 stationary bicycle. *(Courtesy of Schwinn Bicycle Company, Chicago, IL.)*

replaced with dropped ones. The seat is comfortable (although huge) and has a calibrated post with quick-release handle. It can be replaced with a touring seat. The post adjusts from 1 inch to 10 inches, and a longer post is available.

The XR-7's frame is solidly welded steel. Pedals are ball-bearing, rubber block, with straps. They can be replaced by rattrap pedals and toe clips.

This bike is portable, and you can roll it on the flywheel just like a wheelbarrow.

Tension control is via caliper brakes with brake pads and a

dial-type adjustment. The control box is convenient. However, there are no numbers on the tension dial, and it's not calibrated. The brakes respond immediately to tension adjustments.

The XR-7 comes assembled at your Schwinn dealer, and repairs are done at the same dealer.

The outdoor feeling is very good on this bike, and operation is smooth, comfortable, with no vibrations, no bouncing, and no flex. The XR-7 is a real workhorse: you can stand up to pedal and it doesn't budge.

If you're on a budget, this is the stationary bike for you. All it could use is some kind of calibration on the tension (say 0 to 10), so you could repeat your workout the next day.

The 1984 model is the XR-8. Its only differences are the frame design, which, according to the manufacturer, makes it 1.8 times more rigid than the XR-7. The seat height mechanism was also changed—it now consists of a threaded pin that screws into holes on the post. The chain has been replaced with a better-quality one, to reduce the XR-8's noise level.

Schwinn has plans for a smaller version of this bike, designed for apartment use, which you might want to ask about.

Bicycle Ergometers

The word "ergometer" comes from the Greek words "ergon" (work) and "metric" (measurement) and means, obviously, "measurement of work." A bicycle ergometer is different from a stationary bike because an ergometer precisely measures the amount of work you're doing. In fact, many manufacturers claim laboratory accuracy for their ergometers, provided that the calibration is correct. An ergometer allows you to plan your exercise program to duplicate a workload exactly and to calculate your calorie consumption during your workout.

The price range and measurement ability of bicycle ergometers is broad. The cheapest one described here is $440, the most expensive $20,000. Most of them, however, are under $1,000. In this price range you'll find sturdily built, precisely calibrated ergonometric bikes. When you spend more than $1,000, you'll get a bike programmed with microcomputers which can provide a digital readout of everything from your heart rate to calorie consumption during your workout. The $20,000 system includes an oversized television with a video player that takes you on simulated tours of secluded roads.

Unless you have a specific medical problem and your doctor recommends a particularly expensive ergometer, there's little reason to spend over $600.

Unfortunately, it's not as easy to rent an ergometer as to rent a stationary bicycle. They are relatively new on the market, so there hasn't yet been much of a demand. However, it's advisable to at least test ride the ergometer of your choice at a bike store, to be sure that it meets your needs. Sometimes, however, you might even have trouble finding ergometers to test ride. During the summer of 1983, I couldn't find Schwinn's Bio-Dyne or Bodyguard's 955 anywhere in St. Louis and had to have them shipped from the manufacturer.

Each ergometer recommended here was rated on the same characteristics as those used for stationary bikes, plus the following:

- Ease of calibration of workload and ease of recalibration after you've added thousands of miles to the bike.

- Tension control mechanism. In ergometers, this varies from caliper brakes to fabric belts to hydraulic and electronic systems. Also, find out how the workload will be measured. On some ergometers, the workload is recorded in watts. Others use kiloponds, still others kilopond-meters per minute. Some even measure your workload in horsepower or newtons. Your workload increases dramatically when you pedal faster. The best ergometers calculate your workload at different cadences or revolutions per minute (rpms). Most of the time, you'll find it more comfortable, and easier on your joints, to work between 70 and 90 rpm. (See Chapter 5 for more information on cadence.) When you're evaluating the tension control mechanisms on ergometers, remember that this is the feature for which you're paying extra. The controls should be quickly readable, accurately calibrated, and easy to reach.

One group of researchers studied the differences when legs only are trained, compared to when arms *and* legs are trained on a bicycle ergometer such as Schwinn's unusual Air-Dyne. Eleven men followed a fitness program on ergometers, training three times a week. Those who used both their arms and legs did more work at a lower heart rate. The researchers concluded that considerably *less* physical stress was placed on the heart and muscles when arms and legs were *both* used. They suggest that ergometers that encourage both arm and leg exercise be part of the rehabilitation program for cardiac patients.

ERGOMETERS UNDER $600

All ergometers are arranged alphabetically by manufacturer's name. All are of approximately equal quality—read each description for individual variations.

Bodyguard/J. Oglaend 957 Triathlon Trainer ($440).   This is a sturdy, well-made Norwegian model, shown in Figure 3–5. The frame is steel, with solid welding. It comes with a one-year warranty on parts, lifetime on frame. The weight is 60 pounds, and the noise level is low—an advantage if you live in an apartment with paper-thin walls. Leveling feet are not available.

The speedometer registers from 0 to 30 kilometers, and the odometer also reads in kilometers. It's not resettable. Cadence readings of 50, 60, and 70 rpm are noted on the dial. Workload is calibrated from 50 to 250 watts, but only at a cadence of 50 rpm. Ask your dealer (or the distributor) for a paste-on chart that will tell your watts at high pedaling speeds. You can also purchase a metal attachment for the tension control lever that gives your reading in watts at 50, 60, and 70 rpm. The flywheel is solid steel and weighs 30 pounds, although it's not as large as a normal bicycle wheel.

The handlebars, which are quick-release, are adjustable forward and back, as well as up and down from 42 inches to 45 inches. The saddle is of hard plastic, but quite comfortable. The seatpost is not calibrated, but is quick-release. The post adjusts from 30 inches to 41 inches.

Tension is controlled by a nylon friction strap on the flywheel. A built-in gauge allows you to check calibration accuracy, which

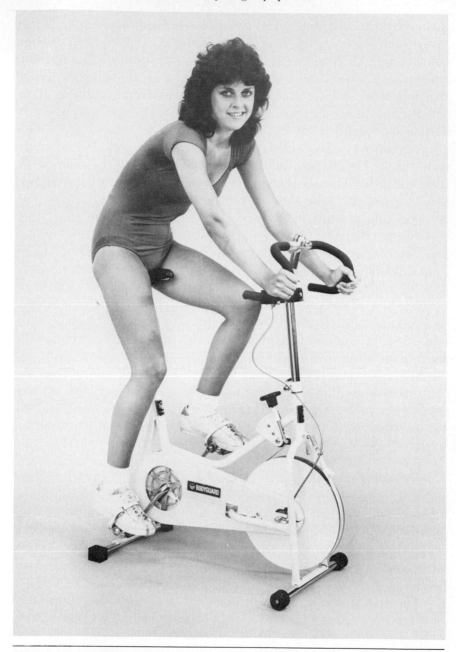

Figure 3–5 Bodyguard 957 Triathlon trainer ergometer. *(Courtesy of J. Oglaend, Inc., Mt. Kisco, NY.)*

is also checked at the factory. An instruction booklet explains the exceptionally easy procedure for checking the tension on a spring. There's a quick response to any tension adjustment. The tension dial on this bike is too low, however; it's a strain to reach down and adjust it. A longer dial would be a welcome addition. The bell-ringing timer and speedometer are easy to reach and to read. Pedals are rattrap with leather straps.

Assembly is easy and took me only 20 minutes. Instructions come in six languages, including English, French, German, and three Scandinavian languages (but not Spanish, unfortunately). You can roll this bike around on the front wheels.

You might want to ask your dealer for a calorie chart (it's accurate at 50 rpm).

This bike is very comfortable, attractive, and easy to ride. Your workout will resemble outdoor riding quite a bit. There is no flex, and no rattles or jerks.

The bike is available from dealers throughout the United States, or you can order through J. Oglaend. Call them toll-free at 800-828-1186. A new workload scale, with smaller increments, will soon be available.

My only suggestions would be to add leveling feet, to reduce the unstable feeling that you have when you sit way back on the seat (their more expensive ergometer has this feature), and to extend the length of the tension control lever so that it's easier to reach.

Monark/Universal Fitness Mark II Ergometer 865 ($450).   This Swedish bike is Monark's entry into the lower-priced ergometer market, and the Mark II is the most popular model for home use. It comes with Universal Fitness's standard warranty of one year on all parts. The Mark II weighs 75 pounds, and it's easy to move when you roll it on the flywheel and small front wheels (see Figure 3–6).

The speedometer reads in kilometers, as does the odometer. No resettable odometer is available. The workload is calibrated in watts with dials accurate for 50 and 60 rpm *only*. You can check the accuracy of the workload measuring device with a 4-kilogram weight. There's also a 30-minute windup timer.

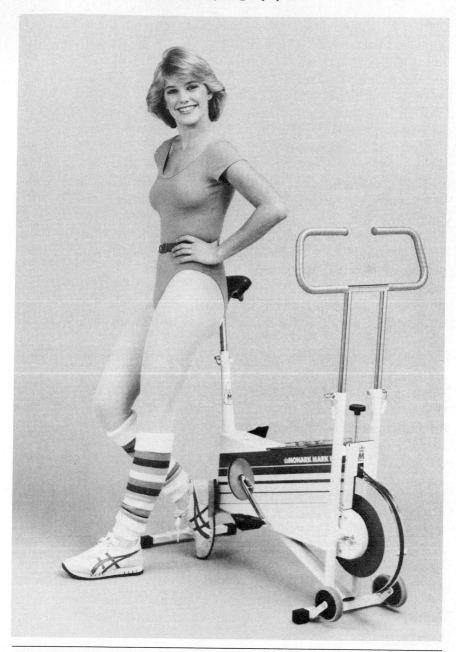

Figure 3–6 Monark Mark II 865 ergometer. *(Courtesy of Universal Fitness Products, Plainview, NY.)*

The Mark II's flywheel weighs 43 pounds and is made of solid steel, as is the frame. A nylon strap provides the tension, and the dial is very responsive to adjustments.

Foam-covered handlebars are adjustable to virtually any position (a new feature on the Mark II that's not shown in Figure 3–6) and they're quick-release. Length adjusts from 33 inches to 49.2 inches.

The oversized soft seat can be replaced with a touring style (an option when you order the Mark II). The post has 13 holes, each one an inch apart, is quick-release, and is "guaranteed no-slide." The post adjusts from 29.5 inches to 42 inches and is 435 millimeters long.

The Mark II's pedals are plastic ball-bearing without toe clips or straps, and are somewhat flimsy. They can be replaced with rattrap pedals and toe clips.

Universal has a toll-free number for repairs (800-645-7554). They have dealers in some states who do repairs, you can buy spare parts and do it yourself, or you can ship the bike back to them.

This ergometer, like all Monarks, is very sturdy and strong, with no bounce, jiggle, or sway.

It's a shame, however, that it is calibrated only for two relatively low cadence levels. Many indoor cyclists prefer to cycle at 70 to 90 rpm, speeds which aren't an option on this bike.

Schwinn/Excelsior Air-Dyne AD-2 ($595).   The Air-Dyne, shown in Figure 3–7, has a unique, patented design that's never been copied. The original design, in fact, came from an Australian company. The workload measurement is also different from other bikes. This is the *only* indoor bike that gives your arms and shoulders a good workout.

This bike comes with the standard Schwinn lifetime warranty, and a free 30-day checkup is included. The Air-Dyne weighs 72 pounds and is cumbersome to move around. It's also one of the noisiest bikes rated here, especially when you close the metal covering over the fan blades.

The Air-Dyne continues Schwinn's reputation for solid, extremely well-built exercise bikes. Its flywheel is composed of a series of "vanes" that turn and produce a fanlike effect on your

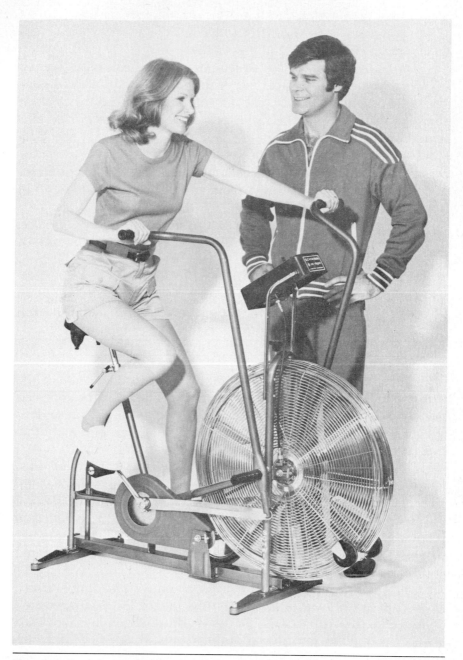

Figure 3–7 Schwinn/Excelsior Air-Dyne AD-2 ergometer. *(Courtesy of Schwinn Bicycle Company, Chicago, IL.)*

legs. As you pedal, the Air-Dyne's arms also move back and forth. When you work both your legs and arms, you increase the fitness level you'd achieve with your legs only.

This bike has leveling feet and an extremely stable base. There's no speedometer, just a tachometer that gives rpm as well as your workload (which, on this bike, is correlated directly with your rpm). In other words, the faster you cycle, the more workload is added by the Air-Dyne's fan.

The timer is digital and battery operated. It shows elapsed or remaining time, and has a 10-second warning beep. The odometer and speedometer both measure in miles, and the odometer is resettable.

Handlebars are obviously not adjustable, since they're a moving part of the bike. They're not quick-release and cannot be replaced.

The saddle is large, but it can be replaced with a racing-style seat (which, however, the manufacturer says might put you in an uncomfortable position). The seat post is calibrated, adjusts from 1 inch to 10 inches, and is quick-release. A longer post is also available.

The cranks are special three-piece eccentric versions that move rather like those on a steam locomotive. Pedals are ball-bearing, rubber block, without toe clips and straps. They can't be replaced due to the unusual crank action. Other pedals might cause dangerous interference with the eccentric cranks, says the manufacturer.

The tension control is a patented "self-regulative air resistance" system. The Air-Dyne is the *only* bike that uses this system. The dial's scale is from 1 to 7 and matches your rpm (this is the only bike to do this). Multiply those six numbers by 300 to calculate your workload in kilopond-meters per minute. The tachometer serves as the workload indicator, and the Air-Dyne is calibrated at all rpm values.

Calibration is checked at the factory, and you can double-check at 50 rpm and a load of 3. It's accurate at sea level, and a scale's included so that you can adjust the readings if you live above sea level. If your bike has calibration problems, your Schwinn dealer will adjust it.

Assembly is at your local Schwinn dealership.

An optional wind screen for the flywheel is available, in case you prefer not to have continual wind blowing on you. Schwinn also has a reading stand especially designed for the Air-Dyne.

Many people are ardent enthusiasts of this bike, including some triathletes. It does give your arms and shoulders (an area that most people don't exercise sufficiently) a terrific workout.

Give the Air-Dyne a try if you think you'd like its unique design. It's a lot of fun to test ride, and the upper body exercise is marvelous.

Schwinn/Excelsior Bio-Dyne BD-1 ($495). The Bio-Dyne is a very sturdy, well-made ergometer (see Figure 3–8). Like all Schwinns, it comes with a lifetime guarantee. A free 30-day checkup is included.

The Bio-Dyne weighs 65 pounds, and its noise level is low to medium. A new chain on the latest models should reduce its noise even more.

Its base is extremely stable and has leveling feet. The speedometer measures in miles per hour, and the odometer calculates miles (of your current trip as well as cumulative). It's resettable.

A tachometer-like monitor on the speedometer indicates your cadence in three ranges only: 60, 75, and 90 rpm. If you want to cycle at 90 rpm (a pace I prefer, as do many indoor cyclists), then this is the ergometer for you.

The Bio-Dyne's timer is digital, with a battery that lasts about a year. You "count down" your time in minutes and seconds, and you can ride as long as 99 minutes, 99 seconds!

The flywheel is an all-metal inertia wheel, and the frame is solidly welded. Handlebars adjust up and down, forward and back, and are easily replaced with dropped bars using the quick-release adjustment.

The seat is huge but easily replaced. The seat post is marked and adjusts easily via a quick-release lever. The post raises from 1 inch to 10 inches, with a longer post available.

The Bio-Dyne's control box is convenient, and it's easy to reach and to read all dials. Pedals are ball-bearing rubber blocks with straps and are easily replaced.

Outdoor feeling is excellent with the Bio-Dyne, and its op-

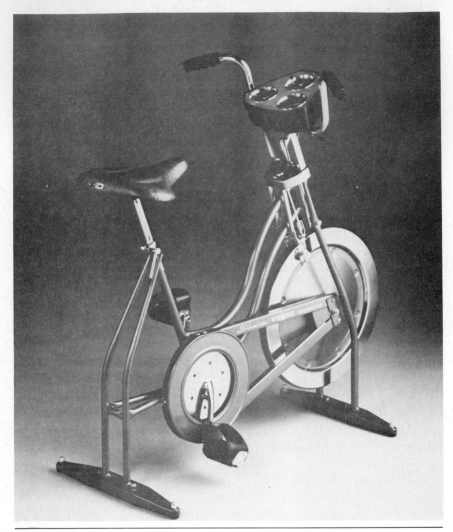

Figure 3–8   Schwinn/Excelsior Bio-Dyne BD-1 ergometer. *(Courtesy of Schwinn Bicycle Company, Chicago, IL.)*

eration is smooth and steady. The bike is portable, since it rolls on the flywheel like a wheelbarrow.

Tension is controlled by hydraulics, with a "Prony" brake resistance system. The Bio-Dyne is calibrated at the factory, and you can purchase a kit to check the calibration. A University of Arizona study found the Bio-Dyne "essentially on calibration" when compared with the Monark 868 and Tunturi 194T.

The Bio-Dyne is assembled at your local Schwinn dealership, and all repairs and adjustments are done there.

This ergometer can be set up by the dealer so that the control box is in a lowered position, but I don't recommend it because there won't be enough room for your hands to rest comfortably on top of dropped handlebars.

ERGOMETERS OVER $600

Ergometers in this category are arranged by price, then alphabetically by manufacturer when prices are the same. The cost of these bikes makes them of limited interest to the general public.

If you have special physical problems, you might want to share this book with your doctor and/or physical therapist so that they can help you decide which ergometer would best meet your needs.

Monark/Universal Fitness Ergometer 868 ($675). A real workhorse, this ergometer, shown in Figure 3–9, was developed with the College of Physical Education in Stockholm, Sweden. World record holders, such as Lon Haldeman and Susan Notorangelo, train on it. It's the bike you frequently see at YMCAs or fitness centers, and you might even have taken a stress test on one.

The Monark 868 comes with the Universal Fitness standard warranty of one year on parts. It weighs 70 pounds and can be moved by rolling it on the flywheel and two small front wheels. No leveling feet are provided.

The speedometer and odomoter read in kilometers, and one odometer is resettable. The tachometer shows rpm from 0 to 130. There's no timer.

The 868's heavy flywheel is made of solid aluminum. Tension is created by a nylon strap on the large flywheel and is measured in newtons and kiloponds. A conversion scale allows you to cycle at any rpm rating. Your workload is calibrated with a 4-kilogram weight, which you'll need to check periodically.

Handlebars are adjustable up and down, forward and back, and are quick-release. Bars extend from 39 inches to 42.5 inches.

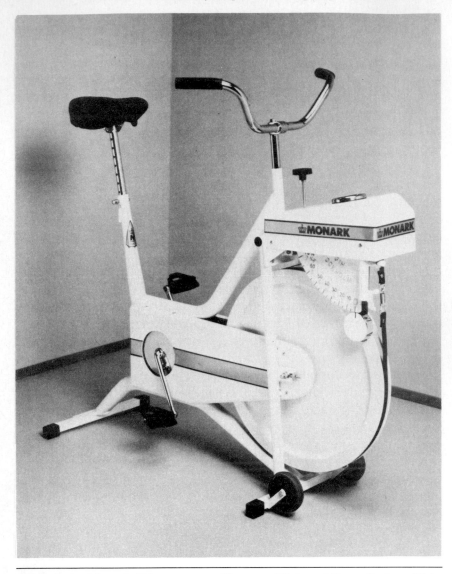

Figure 3–9   Monark 868 ergometer. *(Courtesy of Universal Fitness Products, Plainview, NY.)*

The seat is overstuffed but can be replaced with a touring saddle. It's also quick-release and can be adjusted from 31.5 inches to 44 inches. The seat post is calibrated with holes and is 435 millimeters long.

The chain is protected, and the ball-bearing pedals are plastic, without toe clips or straps.

The frame on this bike is very strong and very stable, with no bounce or flex. It's also relatively quiet.

Universal has a toll-free number for repairs (800-645-7554). They have dealers in some states who do repairs, you can buy spare parts and do it yourself (except, perhaps, for the tension mechanism), or you can ship the bike back to them.

Bodyguard/J. Oglaend Ergometer 990 ($750). This is the more sophisticated version of the Norwegian Bodyguard 957, and it comes with J. Oglaend's standard one-year warranty on parts, lifetime on frame. It's used by the U.S. Olympic Committee for testing and training athletes.

The 990 is heavy (98 pounds) but can be moved around with the large rolling wheels on the front. The crossbar serves as a step when mounting, and is padded with rubber so that it won't get scuffed (see Figure 3–10). The 990 has "level adjusters" (leveling feet).

The speedometer reads in kilometers, as does the odometer. Calibration of the speedometer is done at the factory, and you can check it by the stroboscopic black-and-white scale on the fly-wheel. You also can check the tachometer this way. The 990 has two odometers, one of which is resettable. The 60-minute timer has a bell.

This ergometer's frame is "heavy, solid steel," as is the flywheel, which weighs 29 pounds.

Tension is controlled by a nylon friction strap on the flywheel and a dial lever. Workload goes up to 300 watts, and a chart attached to the control box shows your workload for cadences of 50, 60, and 70 rpm. You "easily" calibrate the bike with a 2-pound weight, according to the distributor. The workload scale is pendulum-like.

Handlebars are dropped, although not in the typical dropped configuration but one unique to Bodyguard. They're adjustable to 360° and can be raised from 40 inches to 48 inches. They're quick-release, with light plastic padding.

The seat is now a plastic racing type, different from the one shown in the photo. The post is calibrated with seven holes, and

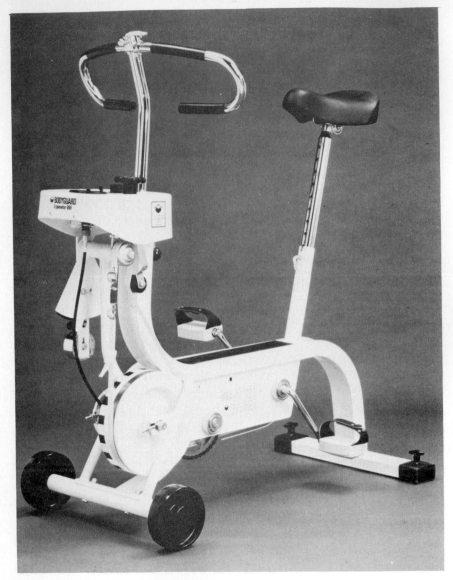

Figure 3–10   Bodyguard 990 ergometer. *(Courtesy of J. Oglaend, Inc., Mt. Kisco, NY.)*

an optional longer seat post is available. The post is quick-release, locks with a locking pin, and adjusts from 26 inches to 40 inches.

The 990's leveling feet make this bike steadier than the 957 (see the section on ergometers under $600). Standard pedals are ball-bearing, made of rubber with straps, but they're easily replaced. If you order rattrap pedals with your 990, they'll be shipped separately and you'll return the originals for credit.

This ergometer is available from dealers throughout the United States, or you can order through J. Oglaend. Call them toll-free at 800-828-1186. Be sure to ask for their calorie chart.

Assembly takes about 5 minutes longer than the 955—so figure about a half-hour. You can perform your own repairs or take the 990 to any bike shop.

Schwinn/Excelsior Electronic Ergometer EX-2 ($1195). This ergometer, shown in Figure 3–11, is Schwinn's top-of-the-line model. It comes with their standard lifetime warranty, as well as a free 30-day checkup.

The frame and base are the same as Schwinn's Bio-Dyne and XR-7, and are equally sturdy and stable, with leveling feet. The EX-2 weighs 85 pounds, and the flywheel is a "deluxe, all-metal inertia wheel."

The EX-2's speedometer measures in miles, as does the odometer. The odometer is resettable. A timer measures in minutes and seconds, up to 60 minutes.

Tension control on the EX-2 is different from the other Schwinns, since it's electronic. Your cycling movements drive a Motorola ac alternator which produces electricity. The amount of current you generate is based on your rpm level.

Eleven settings in kilopond-meters per minute (kpm/min) and in horsepower are marked on the workload indicator in nine increments. The bike's workload measurements are accurate between 50 and 90 rpm, and you *must* pedal at least 50 rpm to get the system to work. Using the load selector switch, you choose the load against which you'll be working. At low speeds, the torque is increased; at high speeds, it is decreased. A built-in speed compensation mechanism holds your workload at a specific kpm/min level no matter how much your cadence varies between 50 and 90 rpm, a nice feature.

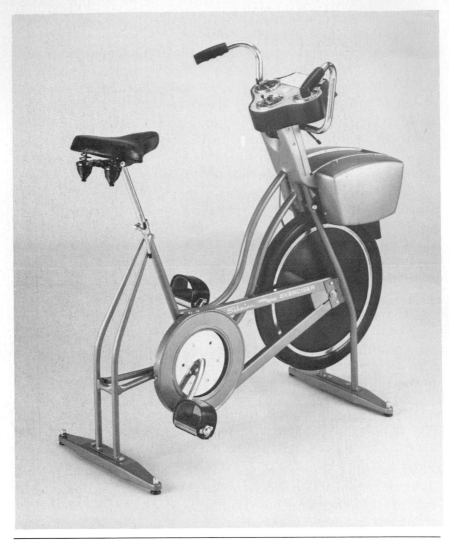

Figure 3–11   Schwinn/Excelsior EX-2 ergometer. *(Courtesy of Schwinn Bicycle Company, Chicago, IL.)*

The EX-2 is calibrated with a dynamometer at the Schwinn plant, and a report of this test comes with the bike.

Handlebars are adjustable up and down, forward and back. They're quick-release, and can be replaced with dropped handlebars.

The seat is large, but it's easily replaced. The post is calibrated, and adjusts from 1 inch to 10 inches. It's quick-release, and a longer post is available.

Pedals are ball-bearing rubber block with straps. You can replace them with no trouble.

The EX-2 can be moved by rolling it like a wheelbarrow. Assembly, repairs, and recalibration are done at the Schwinn dealership.

Extras include a load chart and a score pad with log sheets that's attached to the control panel.

A new EX-3 model will be available sometime in 1985. I'd like to see some way to transfer the electricity you generate to a storage battery of some kind so that you could reduce your home electric bill!

Lifecycle ($1995). This is a heavy bike, at 110 pounds (see Figure 3–12), and it's now the "hot" exercise bike at health clubs. In fact, many clubs charge an additional membership fee for the privilege of using a Lifecycle.

On this steel and plastic bike, you start pedaling, then press the start button to commence the electronic wizardry. You choose a time and exercise level at which you wish to work. A "hill profile" shown on the control box "visually represents terrain encountered in standard programs." It includes warm-up and cool-down segments as well as a series of steady-state and interval workouts.

The Lifecycle's control box shows the calories used per hour and your rpm. It also has an "LED (light-emitting diode) matrix display" that "provides graphic display of present and upcoming effort levels," a timer that shows elapsed time, and a button you press to estimate your maximum oxygen uptake. Your workload is programmed by *calories* on the Lifecycle, which you convert to standard work measurements by using the instruction book.

Your pedaling generates the electricity necessary to run the control box. The manufacturer says that your workload remains constant from 1 to 199 rpm.

The console can be removed if repairs to the bike or to electronic circuits are necessary, although it's difficult when using the Lifecycle at home to determine if the calibration is correct.

The seat is steel with a rubber cover and adjusts to a range of

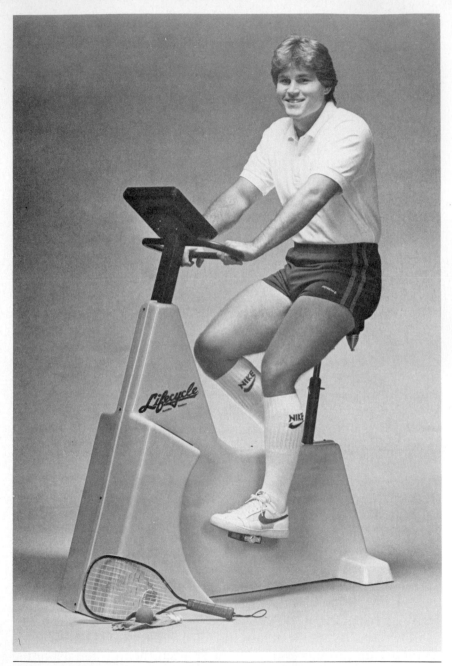

Figure 3–12   Lifecycle ergometer. *(Courtesy of Lifecycle, Inc., Irvine, CA.)*

about 2 feet via a pin-through-a-hole mechanism. The pedals are rubber and can be replaced with rattrap and toe clips. The painted steel handlebars cannot be adjusted at all, since they're built into the control box unit. The manufacturer says that you can add padding, however.

Workloads can be programmed from 300 to 2400 kilometers per minute on this bike, and it has a tachometer. There's no speedometer or odometer on the Lifecycle—a disadvantage if you want to compare your indoor cycling with an on-the-road trip.

The modular electronics unit can be removed and returned to the factory if there's a problem, and it'll be returned within 24 hours of receipt, the manufacturer says.

The Lifecycle comes with a one-year limited warranty on parts and labor. The bike is shipped from the factory by truck, and, once you receive it, you can roll it around on two front wheels.

Monark/Universal Fitness Electronic Ergometer 869 ($1995). This bicycle, shown in Figure 3–13, is exactly the same as the Monark Ergometer 868 described earlier except that a microcomputer has been attached to the 868's body. Included on the console is a tachometer with an audible metronome so that you can keep time with the cadence you're trying to match. A light flashes, as well, if preprogrammed. You receive a digital readout of resistance in newtons, kilopond-meters per minute, or watts. The manufacturer says that it's "easy to calibrate."

You can program your weight, sex, and age, as well as heart rate. An alarm will sound if you're over or under your heart's target zone. You also receive a readout of your pulse, time elapsed, calories consumed, maximum oxygen uptake, and electrocardiogram (ECG) output.

This ergometer comes with Universal Fitness's standard one-year warranty on parts. They also have a toll-free number for repairs (800-645-7554).

Biocycle/Engineering Dynamics Corporation ($2795). The latest entry to the growing computerized indoor cycle market is the Biocycle, shown in Figure 3–14. The manufacturer, Engineering Dynamics Corporation, has produced hospital-grade ergometers for years. This technical proficiency, coupled with a liberal dose

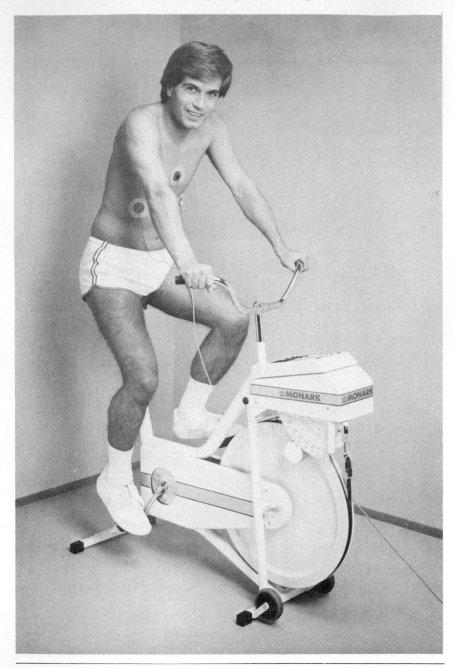

Figure 3–13   Monark 869 electronic ergometer. *(Courtesy of Universal Fitness Products, Plainview, NY.)*

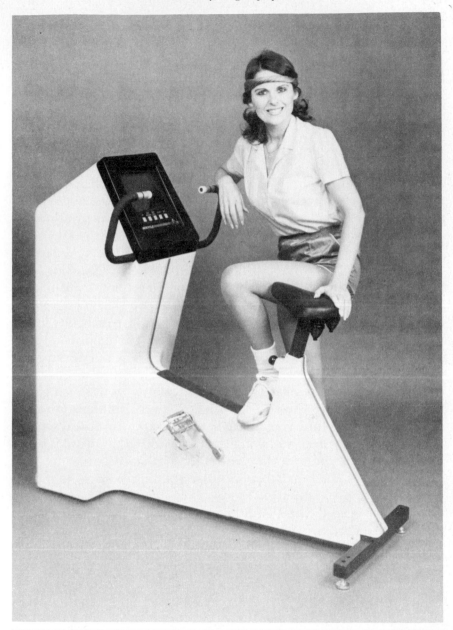

Figure 3–14 Biocycle ergometer. *(Courtesy of Engineering Dynamics Corporation, Lowell, MA.)*

of creativity, has produced an exercise bike that's a lot of fun to ride.

You can choose three sets of programmed "tours" with this bike. First are ten standard program "profiles"—with names like "New England hills," "Rocky Mountain ride," "Surfside beach run," "Boston marathon" (which lasts 24 minutes), and "Olympic bike trials."

The second set of programs allow you to design two original ones of any shape or length. These can be changed whenever you wish. The final program lets you program in the heart rate at which you wish to exercise. The Biocycle then automatically adjusts your workload to maintain that heart rate and continually adjusts the load throughout your workout. (There are extra costs for the second and third groups of programs.)

Other special features include a simulated electrocardiogram-like pulse that helps you "visualize" your heart rate, and twelve levels of difficulty to meet the needs of everyone from beginning to highly advanced riders. By combining the twelve difficulty levels with the ten program profiles, you can create a tremendous variety of workouts.

The video display offered on the Biocycle is full of information, including your pulse, pedal rpm, calories you're using per hour, total calories you've used so far, speed (miles per hour), distance traveled, time remaining in the workout, a "fitness score," the program's profile, and your location within that profile. Your heart rate is monitored via sensors in the handlebar grips. For extra accuracy (such as when you use the target heart rate program), you can wear a chest strap.

The seat is adjustable, and the pedals are rattrap with toe clips. Leveling feet are provided, as is a feature that allows you to bolt the bike to the floor. Although the Biocycle weighs 200 pounds, the manufacturer says that it can easily be rolled around on the front wheels.

This bike comes with a one-year warranty on mechanical and electronic parts, 90 days on the video monitor. Ask the manufacturer about other special program profiles.

Perceptronics/Neiman-Marcus LaserTour Lifecycle ($20,000).   This system combines the Lifecycle ergometer with the LaserTour, a microcomputer with laser videodisc that includes a television screen and a 45-inch rear-screen video projector (see Figure 3–15). You can obtain readouts on your movement speed, terrain changes, and choose your routes via road signs. If you pedal faster or slower, the landscape projected on the screen goes by faster or slower.

You can take various "fantasy tours": Try cycling on a roller

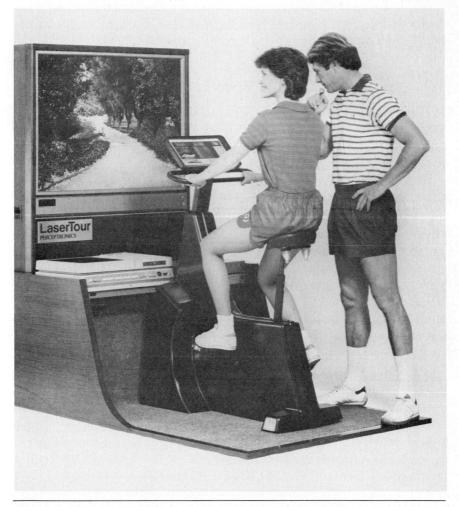

Figure 3–15 Perceptronics/Neiman-Marcus LaserTour Lifecycle. *(Courtesy of Neiman-Marcus, Dallas, TX.)*

coaster or meandering through southern California's scenic back roads. You shift gears via a pushbutton system that the manufacturer says is similar to shifting a 10-speed bike. Approximately two hours of tours currently are available.

You can use the videodisc and television screen without the ergometer, too, and the system will also take videocassettes. Presumably you could tape local tours, then view them while you ride. The Lifecycle can also be used alone.

This unusual, and expensive, system was created especially for Neiman-Marcus. However, Perceptronics is working on a similar, but less expensive, general consumer model.

Wind-Load Simulators and Rollers

Wind-load simulators and rollers are designed to be used with the 10-speed bicycle you already own. Most people who purchase wind-load simulators (WLS) or rollers are outdoor bicycle tourists or racers. They prefer the outdoor feeling of these two types of indoor bicycling equipment, since they can ride their own 10-speed bikes instead of adapting to a stationary bike or ergometer.

Many owners of these two systems ride outdoors as much as they can, then use their WLS or rollers as a backup system or to stress their body in ways that nearby terrain cannot.

One racer from Champaign-Urbana, Illinois, a college town surrounded by flat cornfields, says he "misses the hills" of St. Louis, his former home. He uses his WLS to simulate those hills, and believes that training on the WLS is vital, both to anticipate races in less flat areas of the country and to keep his heart and muscles in fine tone.

If you enjoy cycling outdoors, but find that job schedules or family commitments prevent you from cycling on the road as much as you'd like, perhaps a WLS or a set of rollers is for you.

Wind-load simulators are a relatively new invention, yet in just a few years they have virtually taken over the market segment previously monopolized by rollers.

Although rollers and WLSs cost about the same ($100 to $200), a WLS doesn't force you to learn the complex balancing tasks required by rollers. And many people feel that a WLS more closely approximates the feeling of riding outdoors than do rollers. In addition, with a WLS you can adjust the tension, whereas on rollers you can only plan a fitness program that is as difficult as your gears allow. With a WLS's precise, measurable, reproducible tension, however, your workout more closely resembles that of an ergometer—and a WLS costs considerably less than an ergometer.

Some models of rollers, however, now feature attachments that allow you to increase or decrease tension. In addition, there are now rollers, such as Kreitler's system, that come with a complicated set of attachments that include a fan, speedometer, odometer, tension control, and even a bracket into which you place your bike's front fork after removing the front wheel. A system such as Kreitler's provides the benefits of both rollers and a WLS, and you can choose whether you practice your balance or not, as your mood dictates.

Dr. Ed Burke of the U.S. Cycling Federation compared rollers with a Racer-Mate WLS to determine which type of equipment gave the better workout and whether a cyclist received a "training effect" from each system. Testing at the same three gear ratios, he found that mean heart rates on the rollers were 66, 70, and 76 percent of maximum, while the Racer-Mate averaged 72, 84, and 97 percent with the same gearing. In addition, maximum oxygen consumption varied from 40 to 50 percent on the rollers, while on the Racer-Mate consumption was 48 to 85 percent.

Highly conditioned athletes couldn't keep cycling on the Racer-Mate at the 52:13 gear ratio (the most difficult) for more than 5 minutes. Burke concludes that the Racer-Mate stresses a rider *more* than riding rollers without a WLS attachment.

If you decide to purchase either a WLS or rollers, try them before you buy. I recommend that you bring (or ride) your 10-speed bike to a bike shop to test ride either piece of equipment. That way, you'll be sure your bike fits exactly onto the WLS or rollers. Some disreputable bike dealers will give you an $800 bike (a top-of-the-line 10-speed) to try out their equipment, but when you get home you'll find your $200 bike is not as comfortable.

Some bikes don't fit correctly on wind-load simulators. It's impossible to attach the WLS to the bike's frame, since brake or gear cables are anchored there. Other design elements can prevent you from using your bike on a WLS, and some 15-speed or triple-crank bikes also may not fit correctly.

The criteria used to evaluate WLS and rollers rated here are:

- Steel frame?

- Strong, high-quality construction? No flexing or bouncing as you ride? Sturdy on the floor?

- If rollers, are the rollers high-quality mahogany or turned aluminum? Do they roll quietly and smoothly?

- Speedometer?

- Odometer?

- Is tension resistance available? How does it work? Is it strong? Responsive?

- How much does the equipment weigh?

- What's the noise level? (This is an important consideration, since WLS and rollers are among the noisiest indoor bicycling equipment.)

- How long does initial assembly take? After that, how long does it take to get your bike on and off each time you ride? Do you have to use a wrench, or is it a quick-release system?

- Is the system portable? Does it fold up? (This is important if you take the equipment with you when you travel.)

- Does your bike fit correctly on the system? If you plan to share with your spouse or roommate, be sure that he or she also checks the fit.

- If a WLS, does it convert to a repair stand? (This feature could be invaluable when you need to repair your bike.)

- Is the base level? Are the feet adjustable for uneven floors?

- What accessories are available? (One example is a fan that turns by your pedaling.)

- What is the guarantee?

- What's the floor clearance? (If you have shag or thick carpeting, this is an important consideration. Rollers may not turn correctly if there's not enough clearance over a rug. Your back tire could catch if a WLS doesn't have sufficient clearance.)

- If a WLS, can it be used with rollers?

- If rollers, what are the belts made of? Are they strong? Safe? Sturdy? Maintenance-free? Easy to replace if they break?

- If rollers, is a front fork-support attachment available so that you can learn to balance gradually?

- If rollers, is a WLS attachment available?

- If rollers, are steps available for easy mounting and dismounting?

- If rollers, is the wheelbase adjustable? Does it fit your bike correctly?

- If rollers, are they "dished"? (This means that the middle of each drum is slightly smaller than the edges, which helps you balance at the center of the rollers.)

WIND-LOAD SIMULATORS

Racer-Mate pioneered the idea of wind-load simulators. They introduced their Original Racer-Mate in 1978. Other manufacturers modified similar designs to produce somewhat different models, although the basic principles remain pretty much the same.

If you plan to purchase a wind-load simulator, I'd suggest you buy either a TurboTrainer or a Racer-Mate. Both are high-quality pieces of equipment, and both are available at bike stores throughout the country or by mail order. My discussion is arranged alphabetically.

Racer-Mate. The Original Racer-Mate, invented by chief engineer Wilfried Baatz, placed the caged fans at the very top of the bicycle's rear wheel (Figure 3–16). The latest system, the Racer-Mate II (Figure 3–17), places the fans at the base of the rear wheel (like the TurboTrainer). Both Racer-Mates are still available, so you can take your choice.

Mike Kolin, coach of Seattle's Rainbow Cycling Club, uses the

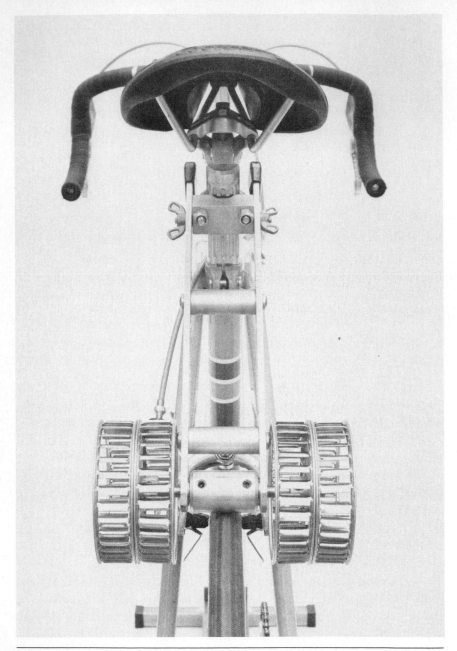

Figure 3–16   Original Racer-Mate wind-load simulator. *(Courtesy of Racer-Mate, Inc., Seattle, WA.)*

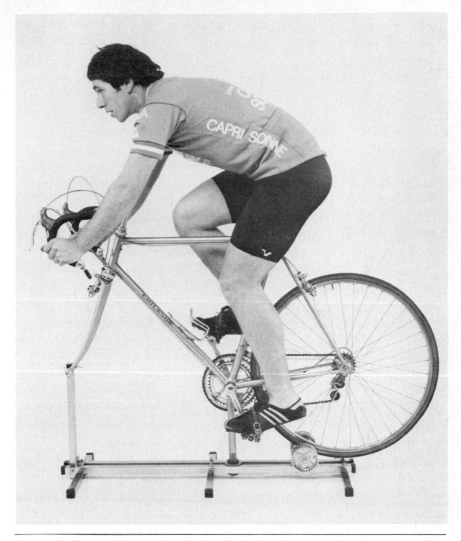

Figure 3–17 Racer-Mate II wind-load simulator. *(Courtesy of Racer-Mate, Inc., Seattle, WA.)*

Racer-Mate extensively with club members. His riders include a number of male and female Olympic-level champions.

One nice feature of the Original Racer-Mate is that, since the squirrel-cage fans are located at the back of your legs, they provide a cooling effect that isn't available from a WLS that has the fans at the base of your wheel.

The Original model allows very little slippage between the cages and your tire. As your speed increases, the cages press harder against the tire, thereby preventing the slippage that occurs with base fans. Thus, the Original model comes very close to achieving the measurement accuracy of a bicycle ergometer.

The Original Racer-Mate is also one of the quietest WLSs you can purchase. The machine's noise is not directly over the floor and slippage doesn't add to the noise level.

Some bicyclists who own rollers without a high enough resistance buy an Original Racer-Mate and add it when they ride the rollers.

The Racer-Mate II has a steel training stand, double-sealed ball bearings, heavy-duty stainless steel shaft, steel tubes, and sturdy crosspieces.

A monitor is now available for the Racer-Mate, on which you can read your workload (in horsepower) and your speed. Simply refer to Figure 5–2, which tells you how many calories you're using, then translate your Racer-Mate speed into equivalent road speed based on your gear. Their chart is extremely helpful for training on this WLS.

Racer-Mates accommodate bikes with cables under the bottom bracket and can even handle triple cranks. However, if you use the Original model, you'll need to remove your fenders or rear carrier before you can attach it.

Assembly of the Racer-Mate is time-consuming (an hour on the average), and reattachment of the Original model each time you ride can also be inconvenient.

A limited warranty of one year is available on both Racer-Mate models. Warranty service is handled on a "same-day" basis.

The Original Racer-Mate, including training stand, sells for a suggested retail of $164.95. Without the stand, it's $91.95. The Racer-Mate II has a suggested price of $119.95, while the monitor sells for $49.95.

TurboTrainer.   Designed by a San Diego racing cyclist, Richard Byrne, this WLS, shown in Figure 3–18, is a sturdy, stable model.

The TurboTrainer is constructed of welded steel, weighs 13 pounds, and can easily be assembled in just a few minutes. There-

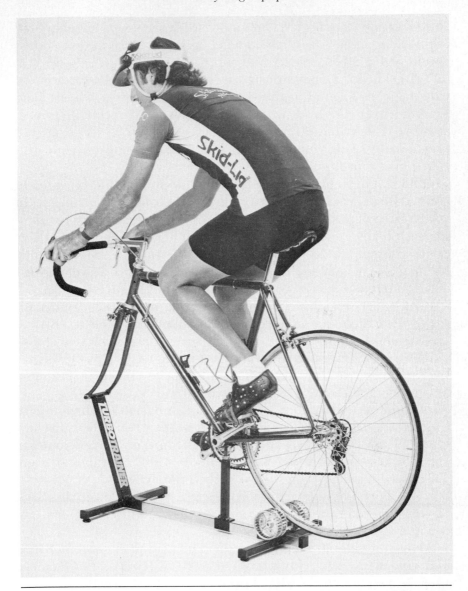

Figure 3–18 TurboTrainer wind-load simulator. *(Courtesy of SkidLid Specialties, Inc., San Diego, CA.)*

fore, you can take it apart and store it if you have a small apartment. Many cyclists take this model on trips to use in their hotel rooms or for a before-race warm-up.

The TurboTrainer's design is quite attractive. The squirrel-cage fans are located at the base of your bike's rear wheel. The manufacturer (SkidLid, which is well known for cycling helmets) says their latest models include a quick-release fork-securing system for the front wheel that enables you to clamp on your 10-speed bike more quickly.

Older TurboTrainer models don't accommodate bikes with control cables under the bottom bracket. However, starting with 1983, TurboTrainer now has a new bottom-bracket support that fits such bikes.

One excellent feature of the TurboTrainer is its adjustable leveling feet, which add tremendously to its stability. Leveling feet are invaluable if you have to ride on an uneven surface.

TurboTrainers have been used by the major velodromes in the United States (a velodrome is a banked bicycling track), including the Olympic Velodrome, by several major bicycle clubs, and by the U.S. Cycling Federation's training facility for the Olympic bicycling team. The team's support vehicles use TurboTrainers as a permanent part of their equipment.

In addition, a number of sports medicine facilities throughout the country use TurboTrainers as part of their rehabilitation programs. Many top cyclists and triathletes train on TurboTrainers. Dave Scott, for example, winner of the 1982 Hawaii Ironman Triathlon, regularly rides on a TurboTrainer.

The TurboTrainer can be converted to a bicycle repair stand by moving the fan assembly slightly forward to disengage it from the rear tire.

You can ride all bicycles on the TurboTrainer, except BMX and tandem. If you own a tandem or BMX, contact the factory, since you can special-order TurboTrainer units for those bikes. Bicycles with fenders or rear carriers can be accommodated on the TurboTrainer.

SkidLid offers a one-year limited warranty on parts and labor. The TurboTrainer can be purchased through bike shops all over the United States, and the suggested retail price is $195.

Or Build Your Own. If you're handy with tools, you might want to get a copy of *Mechanix Illustrated*'s March 1984 issue. It features detailed instructions on how to build your own exercise bike stand, which works like a WLS. Their stand is made of oak and is extremely attractive. Should you need extra resistance, you could always add an Original Racer-Mate to your 10-speed bike.

ROLLERS

Rollers have come a long way from the first ones invented. You can now purchase accessories for rollers such as wind-load simulators, fans, speedometers, and odometers—accessories developed so that rollers could compete with wind-load simulators, and also so that your pulse could go high enough to get an aerobic workout.

Learning to ride the rollers is truly a challenge. If you have any doubts about your balancing ability, are too uncoordinated to ride a bike outdoors, or have a physical handicap that affects your balance, then rollers are not for you. Instead, choose a stationary bike, bicycle ergometer, or a wind-load simulator—none of which requires balancing ability.

If you don't do much outdoor bicycling, or haven't ridden a 10-speed bike for many years, you might not want rollers unless they come with a stand to support your bike's front axle. Such a stand serves like "training wheels" did on your first bike. Once you're proficient with the stand, you progress to riding the rollers without it.

But don't immediately decide that your balancing ability is nonexistent. With a little help from a friend, you probably can learn to ride rollers. You'll need someone to hold the back of your saddle while you find a comfortable position. The friend should continue holding on until you're secure balancing alone. It sometimes helps to set your rollers in a doorframe so that you'll have something sturdy to hang on to if you feel yourself slipping.

Try rollers at your bike shop, and ask the sales person to show you how to mount and dismount and teach you the correct balance. Some people pick up the knack in only a few minutes, whereas others (including me) take longer.

In many ways roller-riding is the best preparation for riding outdoors. But rollers are also the most difficult kind of equipment to ride.

Rollers are discussed in alphabetical order.

Kreitler Rollers.   Virtually everyone who rides rollers rates Al Kreitler's system, shown in Figure 3–19, the best.

John Pixton, Chairman of the Bicycling Federation of Pennsylvania, who rides more than 1500 roller-miles a year, has described the Kreitler system as being of superb quality and excellent design. Thom Lieb and Tom Walz, reviewing various rollers for *Bicycling* magazine, concur. Lieb considers the Kreitler rollers the best ones made, and Walz is especially impressed by their silent operation.

Lon Haldeman, holder of the numerous world bicycling records mentioned earlier, has trained on Kreitler rollers, and says they're the best rollers made. He likes the Kreitler rollers and Headwind system "because they give the feeling of riding on the road and the resistance I need."

Kreitler's Headwind blower unit has an air intake damper that you open or close to change the resistance. Of course, you also can change gears to change the difficulty of your workout. A unique feature of Kreitler's Headwind system is that when the damper is open, it acts as a fan to cool you off. Kreitler says that his Headwind system can be used "by a 98-pound weakling or a

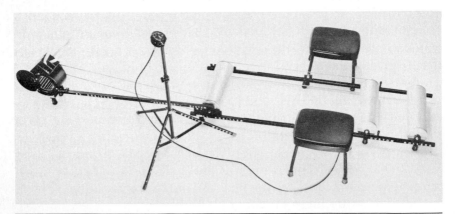

Figure 3–19   Kreitler rollers. *(Courtesy of Al Kreitler, Kansas City, MO.)*

super-athlete like Lon Haldeman. It's tough, but oh, so gentle, if need be." With the Headwind system, you "match your load to your training needs." When the blower is wide open, however, only the very best riders can keep pedaling.

Kreitler rollers come completely assembled, adjusted, and ready to ride. They fold in half and store easily in a closet. These rollers are carefully designed so that they don't bounce at high speeds. Bearings are sealed, and belts are made of polyurethene (which resists breakage better than rubber belts, Kreitler says) and are recessed in the drums. The frame is made of steel tubing.

These rollers are about the quietest available. In addition, a Stewart-Warner speedometer and odometer attachment with an adjustable stand is available. Kreitler says that it's accurate within 1 percent. Steps to make mounting easier are optional. Brand-new items are a bike stand that aids beginners' balance, and a Spin Coach feature that teaches you to use both legs equally.

Kreitler also makes rollers that can be used with tandems and children's BMXs.

In 1983, Kreitler rollers were used to obtain a 24-hour world record for roller-riding (838.6 miles). Kreitler rollers designed for tandem bicycles hold the 24-hour tandem record of 604.0 miles.

These rollers are guaranteed up to five years. Costs for the system are as follows: alloy rollers, $275.00; PVC rollers, $159.95; fork, $39.95; Headwind system, $89.95; speedometer, $74.95; steps, $44.95. Keep in mind that you're paying for excellent workmanship and state-of-the-art technology.

MTD Rollers (Bike Nashbar). MTD's mahogany rollers, distributed by Bike Nashbar's mail-order house, are just beautiful (see Figure 3–20). They are a basic, well-made, sturdy set of rollers, and all parts come with a five-year guarantee.

Handmade and hand-assembled, these rollers feature shielded bearings, sturdy belts, and aluminum side rails with flanges to prevent tire damage. The mahogany drums are lathe-turned for smoothness.

MTD rollers stand upright for storage and fit easily into a closet.

Solid mahogany steps are also available. You can purchase MTD's drums in mahogany, aluminum, or plastic, or in combina-

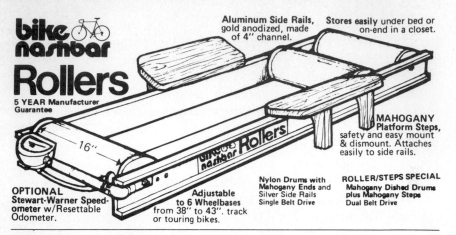

Figure 3–20   MTD rollers. *(Courtesy of Bike Nashbar, New Middletown, OH.)*

tions of plastic and mahogany or aluminum and mahogany. A Stewart-Warner speedometer is available for these rollers.

John Pixton, writing in *Bicycling* magazine, rated the MTD rollers a best buy. Special rollers for children's BMX bikes are available in plastic and mahogany.

Assembly takes about a half-hour. The instructions, however, are not in sequence.

If you decide to purchase MTD rollers, you might also buy an Original Racer-Mate to provide the resistance you'll need to produce aerobic benefits.

Suggested retail prices for MTD rollers are: mahogany drums, $225.00; all-aluminum drums, $225.00; aluminum/plastic drums, $179.95; all-plastic drums, $175.43; plastic/mahogany drums, $143.36; speedometer, $25.00; and mahogany steps, $49.95. Bike Nashbar's catalog (see Appendix F) attractively discounts these suggested prices.

4

Invaluable Accessories

Outdoor bicycling has spawned an incredible number of small industries serving cyclists' various needs. Some of the equipment you'd use outdoors, such as a helmet, rain suit, storage bags, and water bottles, aren't necessary for indoor cycling. Other accessories, however, are absolutely essential.

One of these is a set of downturned handlebars. Research has proven that compared to upright handlebars, downturned bars can maximize your work output, increase your lungs' ability to process air, and help you use calories more effectively. Another essential accessory is a racing seat, which enables you to use all the large muscles in your thighs and buttocks. Then there are rattrap pedals with toe clips; these force your feet into the proper position and help you make the best use of those large muscles in the back of your thighs. So plan to add each of these items to your indoor equipment—if they are not provided by the manufacturer—and add the cost of such accessories when you figure the total budget for your setup. I'd suggest that you add these accessories before you leave your bike shop, if possible.

In addition to these basics, you'll want to purchase a powerful fan or two (unless you're using an Original Racer-Mate or riding Schwinn's Air-Dyne); padding for your handlebars (to reduce pressure on the sensitive ulnar nerve that runs through your wrist and branches into your palm); padding for your bike seat or shorts (since saddle sores can be a problem even indoors); and a reading stand (even if you don't want to read, a stand is great for holding records of your progress).

A wristwatch or clock with a second hand are helpful when you're practicing brief, intense intervals, or if your equipment doesn't come with a timer. Many people also keep a cotton towel under their bike or on the frame, since they drip perspiration.

DOWNTURNED HANDLEBARS

If your bike doesn't already come with them, make sure that you purchase a set with plenty of room at the top for your hands (preferably a Randonneur bar). As you ride, vary the position of your hands along the flat top tube, and occasionally move down to the "drops" (the lowest part of the handlebars) when you do "intervals" (see Chapter 5). You'll never regret purchasing dropped handlebars: your rear end will thank you, since by leaning forward you take pressure off it, as will your hands, since you'll have plenty of places to put them should you get bored or stiff in any one position.

Look for handlebars that are about the same width as your shoulders. Get your bike store to recommend a high-quality brand—but it's not necessary to buy the most expensive since you'll experience no road shock. I use Schwinn's basic model, which costs about $15.

RACING SEAT

Seats, however, are another story. The variety of styles are amazing, and this may be the most important accessory you'll ever buy.

Many people quit an indoor cycling program either because of boredom or because of a very sore rear end. To avoid the first problem, see Chapter 8, "Motivational Tips." To avoid the second, get rid of the wide seat that usually comes with your exercise bike. It'll be torture on your thighs after a hundred miles (that's when I threw mine out) and you won't be able to lean forward on your new downturned handlebars without getting a sore rear.

You can choose from leather or plastic "saddles" (as the racers call them) and from a number of new novelty seats designed to reduce friction and soreness.

Breaking in a leather saddle can take a thousand miles or so. If you decide to purchase such a seat, use a saddle pad and/or lots of neatsfoot oil until you and the seat are used to one another. Brooks ($30) is a well-known and highly touted leather saddle.

Most professional cyclists now use padded, leather-covered plastic saddles, such as those made by Turbo, Concor, or Avocet. Expect to pay $15 to $20. Avocet offers different versions for men and women, designed to reflect the anatomical differences between the sexes. Unfortunately, a plastic saddle never breaks in to fit your body's contours as leather will.

The Easyseat, a new-style seat designed so that there's nothing but air between your legs, is made by JB Two. I tried this $20 seat and liked it for about 500 miles. However, I always felt that I was slipping forward onto the pedals, and I apparently wasn't using my hamstring and buttock muscles as much, since my quadriceps got very sore while those other muscles felt unused. I did, however, find that I used my abdominal muscles more (to hold me on the seat, I suppose) and I lost an inch around my abdomen in less than a month! I never felt saddle sores of any kind. Eventually, however, I decided the Easyseat was not for me, and returned to a racing model with padding.

RATTRAP PEDALS WITH TOE CLIPS

If your exercise equipment doesn't already come with rattrap pedals, toe clips, and straps, have your bike dealer remove yours and substitute them. Many varieties are available, and your bike shop dealer can steer you in the right direction. Again, there's no reason to buy the most expensive, since you won't be on the road. Expect to pay a total of $15 to $20.

Toe clips match your shoe size. If you're a woman, it's helpful to know what size you take in a man's shoe, since clips come in men's small, medium, and large.

Have your dealer assemble the pedals and clips, then try them out. For your toes to be completely comfortable, you must have a little room at the end of the clip. The ball of your foot should fit directly on the pedal when your toes are in the clips. Wear the straps as tight or as loose as you want, since you don't have to worry about sudden stops.

Once you're accustomed to using toe clips and straps as part of your indoor cycling program, you'll find that you don't feel right without them outdoors. And you'll realize how much energy you wasted when your feet wandered all over the pedals.

A FAN (OR TWO)

Don't even consider cycling indoors without a fan (or two). If you don't believe me, just try cycling for 30 minutes on your indoor bike in the spring or summer. You'll work up such a sweat that you probably won't be able to finish. With a fan placed in front of your bike to simulate outdoor wind currents, however, you'll be able to pedal almost indefinitely.

Purchase whatever fan appeals to you. If your bike will be placed in front of a window, try a huge window fan (about $25). If you exercise in a hallway or a room with windows that don't open, a large floor fan might be best. I'd suggest that you buy a fan that has three speeds, such as Sears' $90 high-velocity model. It's expensive, but well worth the cost if you don't have air conditioning.

Some people bicycle in front of an air conditioner in the summer, but that gets mighty cold in the winter. If your air conditioner can be switched to a fan setting, try that. If not, you'll probably still need a fan in the winter—unless you plan to open the windows, of course. You'll be surprised at how much heat your body generates when you cycle indoors in the winter.

HANDLEBAR PADDING

Handlebar padding is necessary to reduce excess pressure on the sensitive ulnar nerve in your wrists and hands. When you purchased downturned handlebars, you have to put handlebar tape over the bare metal anyway. Instead, purchase padding, put it on, and cycle comfortably from then on.

I started cycling indoors using plastic handlebar tape. After about 1500 miles, my wrists and elbows began to ache after a workout. Then I added Grab-On's $7 handlebar padding, which worked wonders. I highly recommend it.

You'll also be interested in Spenco's entry in the handlebar market. Their $10 Grips are delightful, and feature "millions of built-in nitrogen bubbles . . . bonded externally with polypropylene, which wicks moisture away from the hands while absorbing no moisture itself." These soft, pliable pads come with an unconditional two-year guarantee, and I also recommend them.

SEAT PADDING

If you've already purchased a racing seat, give it a try. Should you get sore, buy some padding for your seat.

Innovative Spenco has entered the seat padding market. Their $22 saddle pad is about the softest, most comfortable one around. It's made of "a lifelike elastomer which absorbs pressure and shocks to prevent soreness and numbness . . . [it's] covered with weatherproof polypropylene." It has a one-year guarantee, and the manufacturers say that it provides "three times more protection and comfort than . . . other . . . cushioning materials."

Or, if you want style, try the $9 Merino wool seat cover made by Cannondale. It's thick, plush, and very comfortable. It would be difficult to get saddle sores with this comfy cover.

If you've never tried a saddle cover, you'll be amazed at the substantial difference some padding can make in how comfortable your rear end stays.

BICYCLING SHORTS

In addition to padding your saddle, you might want to pad your clothing. A good pair of cycling shorts with high-quality chamois padding costs about $35. A bit expensive, but you can wear them both indoors and when you ride your 10-speed bike outside.

Although I prefer 100 percent cotton clothing, many cyclists don't. You'll find shorts in materials from all-cotton or wool to all-nylon or polyester. You have to decide which is best and most comfortable for you.

Cannondale makes a nice pair of cycling shorts with chamois padding that are comfortable and allow leg room for cycling. They're trim and fit well. If you're also going to wear your shorts outdoors, be sure to get them with pockets.

Should you already have a favorite pair of shorts, you can sew in chamois or acrylic pile padding for less than $10. Bike Nashbar sells both by mail order.

READING STAND

I consider a reading stand an invaluable accessory, since I don't enjoy watching television or listening to my stereo while I cycle. But I do enjoy reading, especially during the less strenuous segments of my workout.

Even if you don't want to read, a reading stand is a terrific place to keep a log that records your progress.

Schwinn makes an excellent sturdy $19 reading stand (see Figure 4–1). It fits virtually all handlebars, but if yours are an unusual diameter, ask your dealer about it.

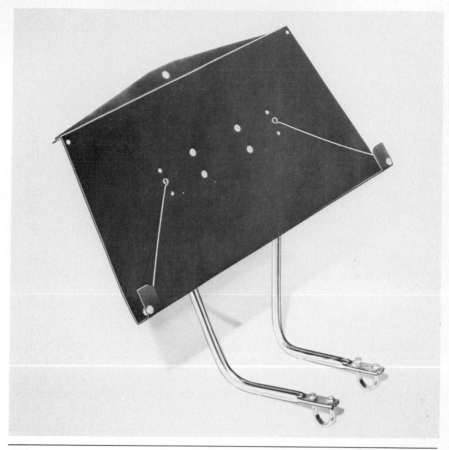

Figure 4–1 Reading stand. *(Courtesy of Schwinn Bicycle Company, Chicago, IL.)*

5

Fitness Programs

This chapter shows you how to design a personalized easy-to-follow fitness program to fit the indoor bicycling equipment you've chosen.

A QUIZ

Before you plan your indoor fitness program, however, be sure to respond to the questions below.[1] No matter what your age, if you answer "yes" to *any* of these questions, you must consult your doctor before you start any indoor bicycling program.

If you're over 35, even if you answered "no" to all the questions, consult your doctor to see if he or she can arrange a bicycle

[1] Reprinted with permission from *Beyond Diet . . . Exercise Your Way to Fitness and Heart Health,* by Lenore R. Zohman, M.D., courtesy of the Mazola Nutrition/Health Information Service.

ergometer stress test for you. Once you've passed 35, you may have heart disease or other physical problems (such as diabetes) without having any outward symptoms. Only a properly administered stress test (coupled with a complete physical exam) can discover such "hidden" problems.

1. Hidden or overt heart disease

    (a) Has a doctor ever said you had heart trouble?

    (b) Have you ever had rheumatic fever, twitching of the limbs called St. Vitus dance, or rheumatic heart disease?

    (c) Did you ever have, or do you now have a heart murmur?

    (d) Have you ever had a real or suspected coronary occlusion, myocardial infarction, coronary attack, coronary insufficiency, heart attack, or coronary thrombosis?

    (e) Do you have angina pectoris?

    (f) Have you ever had an abnormal electrocardiogram or ECG?

    (g) Have you ever had an electrocardiogram taken while you were exercising (such as climbing up and down steps) which was *not* normal?

    (h) Have you ever had pain or pressure or a squeezing feeling in the chest which came on during exercise or walking or any other physical or sexual activity?

    (i) If you climb a few flights of stairs fairly rapidly, do you have tightness or pressing pain in your chest?

    (j) Do you get pressure or pain or tightness in the chest if you walk in the cold wind or get a cold blast of air?

    (k) Have you had bouts of rapid heart action, irregular heart action, or palpitations?

    (l) Have you ever taken digitalis, quinidine, or any drug for your heart?

(*m*) Have you ever been given nitroglycerin, sometimes labeled TNG or NTG, or any tablets for chest pain which you use by placing them under the tongue?

2. Other heart attack risk factors

(*a*) Do you have diabetes, high blood sugar, or sugar in the urine now?—at any time in the past?

(*b*) Have you ever or do you now have high blood pressure or hypertension?

(*c*) Have you been on a diet or taken medications to lower your blood cholesterol?

(*d*) Are you more than 20 pounds heavier than you should be?

(*e*) Has there been more than one heart attack or coronary attack or person with heart trouble in your family before age 60 (blood relative)?

(*f*) Do you now smoke more than a pack and a half of cigarettes per day?

3. Further limiting conditions

(*a*) Do you have any chronic illness?

(*b*) Do you have asthma, emphysema, or other lung condition?

(*c*) Do you get very short of breath on activities which don't make other people similarly short of breath?

(*d*) Have you ever gotten or do you now get cramps in your legs if you walk several blocks?

(*e*) Do you have arthritis, rheumatism, gout or gouty arthritis, or a predisposition to gout? Has the uric acid in your blood been found to be high?

(*f*) Do you have any condition limiting the motion of your muscles, joints, or any part of the body which could be aggravated by exercise?

TYPES OF EXERCISE

I'll refresh your memory on the definitions of two very important terms that refer to exercise. *Aerobic* means with oxygen, and it refers to any form of continual exercise that makes your heart beat more quickly, but where not much painful lactic acid accumulates. *Anaerobic,* in contrast, means without oxygen, and it applies to exercise that you can continue only for a few minutes due to the incredible demands it makes on your heart, lungs, and muscles, as well as the accumulation of painful lactic acid that makes your cells so acidic they fatigue almost immediately.

In any basic fitness program, the aerobic component is *far* more important than the anaerobic. Many people, in fact, follow a fitness program for years and never exercise anaerobically.

The "talk test" is recommended by many sports doctors to determine whether you're exercising aerobically. If you can carry on a conversation without huffing and puffing, you're probably exercising aerobically. If the great gulps of air you're taking keep you from conversing, you're probably exercising anaerobically. You can also check your pulse to determine whether you're exercising in the aerobic range.

There are, however, some training advantages to anaerobic exercise. For example, you can increase your strength and working capacity (measured by the maximum amount of oxygen your lungs consume) with judicious use of anaerobic *sprints* (*intervals*) in a program that's composed primarily of aerobic work.

To create a well-rounded fitness program, all you need to do is combine a basic aerobic workout with a few stretching exercises before and after each workout and some strength-improving exercises. (See Chapter 6 for more details.)

Should you decide to follow a three- or four-day-a-week aerobic program, you could do strength training exercises on alternate days. Don't leave them out, however. The ones recommended here were chosen to work those muscles that otherwise aren't used by indoor bicycling.

You should also stretch *whenever* you ride your bike. If you don't stretch—before *and* after each workout—you're much more likely to have sore muscles, or even pull a muscle. It doesn't hurt to stretch on alternate days, either, perhaps while you watch television in the evenings.

IMPORTANT POINTS
ABOUT AEROBIC EXERCISE

Heart Rate and Target Zone

If you don't monitor your pulse at all times, you're just "spinning your wheels." You have no way to find out whether you're following a heavy workload or a light one. From personal experience, I can tell you that what feels like a "hard" workout for your legs may not be a "hard" workout for your heart. Numerous times my legs have given out when my heart had barely reached my target zone. Now that my leg strength has improved from years of indoor cycling, however, that seldom occurs.

To set up your fitness program, you should plan to work out at a level between 70 and 85 percent of your *maximum heart rate,* a number that can easily be predicted from your age. Take the number 220, then subtract your age from it; that is your maximum heart rate.

Next, you should take 70 and 85 percent of that number (or you can simply use Figure 5–1). This is the *exercise heart rate range* or *target zone* within which you'll want your pulse to stay while you're exercising, to ensure that your workout is aerobic.

This chart, in fact, can be consulted no matter what aerobic sport or activity you participate in. Just remember always to keep your heart rate within the target zone. When you exercise in your target zone for 20 minutes or longer, you know that you're receiving the proper aerobic benefits.

As you age, your maximum heart rate will decrease. Accordingly, your range will also decrease. For example, when you're 50, your range will be 119 to 145 beats per minute, although when you were 30 it was 136 to 165 beats per minute.

Do you know how to take your pulse? It's not difficult. One

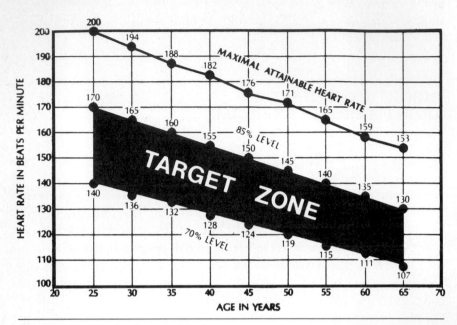

Figure 5–1 Maximal attainable heart rate and target zone. (Reprinted with permission from L. Zohman, M.D., *Beyond Diet: Exercise Your Way to Fitness and Heart Health,* CPC International, Englewood Cliffs, NJ.)

way is to locate your pulse (heart rate) at your wrist. Turn your hand over so your palm is facing you. Then place the two middle fingers of your other hand around your wrist. Press lightly until you find a pulse on the inside of your wrist.

Some people, however, can't easily find a pulse at their wrist. If you're one of them, try taking a reading at the main arteries on your neck. (I find this easier than at the wrist.) Using the same two middle fingers, press lightly on the area of your neck that's just outside your Adam's apple. Don't press too hard (since some people get dizzy from that)—just do it hard enough to locate your heartbeat.

Try to find your pulse now. If you have trouble, try when you've been exercising, since your pulse is *much* easier to find when it's raised above 100.

To calculate your pulse for a minute, take a count for 15

seconds, then multiply that value by 4. If you're not proficient at multiplying while you're exercising, make a copy of the following chart and keep it nearby.

15-Second Count	Beats per Minute
27	108
28	112
29	116
30	120
31	124
32	128
33	132
34	136
35	140
36	144
37	148
38	152
39	156
40	160
41	164
42	168
43	172
44	176
45	180
46	184
47	188
48	192
49	196
50	200

If you need an extremely accurate measure of your pulse (such as when you're under doctor's orders), you might want to invest in one of the heartbeat monitors discussed in Appendix A.

Although heart rate is a reasonably accurate gauge of how hard you're working, many factors affect your pulse. They can include your current physical condition; your general health and emotional state; environmental conditions; how long it's been since your last meal; whether you've had prolonged bed rest; and your amount of body fat.

Monitoring your pulse is especially helpful if you've been sick, in the hospital, or have not been exercising regularly for whatever reasons.

Return to an exercise program slowly and easily. Monitor your pulse at all times. After a layoff, your heart will beat faster at the same workload because you've lost some of exercising's "training effect." However, if you persist at a rate your heart can easily handle, in just a few weeks you'll be almost back at your former fitness level.

You might also want to get into the habit of taking your pulse early in the morning, before you get out of bed. Then you'll be able to watch it *decrease* as you continue your indoor cycling program—which it will.

As your program progresses, in fact, you'll need to make minor changes in your workout based on your pulse on a particular day. You'll find, as I have, that when heat and humidity are both high, your pulse *quickly* reaches the upper limit of your range. However, when it's cool and dry, you'll easily maintain a lower pulse at the same workload. Women often will note variances in their pulse according to what phase of their menstrual cycle they are in, and they should adjust their workload accordingly.

Monitoring your pulse is especially important if you're using a stationary bike or rollers without a tension device, since they don't have any instruments to measure your workload objectively. Therefore, the only measurement you can use to discover how hard you're working is your heart rate.

How Long Should You Exercise?

There's a minimum amount of time you should devote to your aerobic program to produce the desired physical and mental benefits. Experts suggest at least 20 minutes of continuous exercise; 30 minutes is even better.

At the beginning of your fitness program, however, you'll only work about 10 minutes, then you'll gradually increase to 15, later to 20. This gradual pace helps prevent injuries, and is not so overwhelming for the beginner.

You should also spend at least 5 minutes warming up slowly on your bike, and after your program is finished spend another 5 minutes cooling down. You warm up to increase the internal temperature of your muscles and cells. Nerve cells react better after you warm up, so oxygen is more easily transferred to your working muscles. You'll also accumulate less pain-producing lactic acid and your exercising heart rate will be lower than if you start your workout "cold." Some studies found that *without* a warm-up, abnormal changes in the heart can occur and arterial blood pressure can show sudden rises.

Dr. Irwin Faria suggests that light, easy pedaling at the conclusion of your exercise session (the cool-down) gets rid of lactic acid more quickly than if you suddenly dismount. In addition, if you ignore the cool-down, your blood might pool in your legs and you could actually get dizzy or even faint when you suddenly stop exercising.

If you're like most people who commence a fitness program, however, you want to take as many shortcuts as possible. Unfortunately, this is a mistake. If you reduce or eliminate your warm-up and cool-down, you'll run a greater risk of exercise-related injuries, such as muscle strains and tears, as well as that painful accumulation of lactic acid.

If you should end up so sore from your indoor cycling that you don't want to ride again two days later, you're not spending enough time stretching, warming up, and cooling down.

How Often Should You Exercise?

Your basic indoor bicycling fitness program should be practiced, at a minimum, three days each week.

If you want to lose weight on your fitness program, however, you'll eventually want to cycle five or six days a week, since your weekly calorie deficit will be higher that way.

It's not a good idea to exercise seven days a week, though. Your body needs rest. Some studies even indicate that you run a *higher* risk of injury when you exercise seven days a week.

You're also more likely to continue an exercise program and stay motivated if you make it a habit. To do this, try to exercise at the same time every day—perhaps when you get up in the morning, before lunch, immediately after you get home from work, before dinner, or even just before bed (although some people have trouble getting to sleep when they exercise that late).

It makes no difference what time you choose, since the important fact is that you always exercise at the *same* time. Once your bicycling program has become firmly established, you'll feel a vague sense that something's missing if you don't exercise. And once indoor bicycling is a habit and you feel fitter and more alert, you'll probably stay with the program forever.

Cadence

There's a strong relationship between cadence [revolutions per minute of the pedals (rpm)] and the efficiency of your cycling in terms of how much work you produce.

Researchers have found that pedaling at very low speeds (below 50 rpm) and at very high speeds (above 90 rpm) produces higher heart rates and oxygen uptakes than do cadences of between 50 and 90 rpm.

A study reported in *Perceptual & Motor Skills* tested male college students on a bicycle ergometer at rpm rates of 40, 60, and 80. All students cycled at a constant tension level of 840 kilopond-meters per minute (kpm/min). They said their exertion "felt" far *more difficult* at 40 rpm than at 60 or 80. The researcher's data correlated with the students' subjective evaluation, confirming that the subjects' heart rates, oxygen uptakes, and breathing rates actually were higher at 40 rpm.

Research indicates you'll be more comfortable, and your muscles more efficient, if you pedal at least 60 rpm. Many professional cyclists pedal at a considerably higher rate than this—some as high as 90 to 100 rpm, or even more.

The easiest way to measure your cadence (if you haven't purchased a bike computer that calculates it for you) is to count each time your right knee reaches the top of its stroke. Count for 15 seconds. Then convert your 15-second count to rpm, using the chart on the next page.

Many people who commence an indoor bicycling program decide to make it "really hard" by pedaling very slowly at a tension level that's much higher than their muscles are in shape for. This is the *wrong* way to make your program difficult. Why? Because, first, pedaling at a very slow speed is more monotonous than cycling at a higher rpm rate (see Chapter 8 for more details).

15-Second Count	Cadence
10	40
11	44
12	48
13	52
14	56
15	60
16	64
17	68
18	72
19	76
20	80
21	84
22	88
23	92
24	96
25	100
26	104
27	108
28	112
29	116
30	120

Second, when you pedal very slowly with a high tension level, the quadriceps muscles in the front of your thighs might cramp before your heart rate reaches your target zone.

Although you may not be comfortable at 90 rpm when you first start your fitness program, try to maintain at least 50 or 60 rpm from the very beginning. As your condition improves and your legs get stronger, aim for a constant cycling cadence of 70 to 90 rpm. That's not as difficult as it may seem and, in reality, is much *easier* than cycling slowly at high tension levels.

Overload Principle and Plateau Effect

There are two basic principles of exercise physiology with which you should be familiar.

The *overload principle* is a simple but important concept. It says that you must overload a body system (whether it's your muscles or your heart) to improve its physical condition—its fitness.

At first, when your fitness level is low, it's not difficult to "overload" your muscles and your heart. Later in your aerobic program, however, you must do *more* work to keep improving your fitness level.

Aerobic programs in this chapter are arranged by week, and they get progressively more difficult. Since your body will gradually adapt to a higher level of work, your program must become progressively more difficult.

After 10 weeks, when you reach the maintenance level, you should still remember the overload principle. Although unlikely, it's possible that your heart may eventually become so fit that your pulse will fall below the lowest level of your target zone. To keep it "overloaded," you'll need to make your maintenance level more difficult. Choose a faster cadence, higher tension, or simply extend your workout time.

The second principle is the *plateau effect*. If you've even been on a diet, you'll immediately recognize this syndrome. What happens? For a while, you'll show great improvement in your fitness (or you'll lost a lot of weight). Then, for no apparent reason, your improvement plateaus—levels off.

Unfortunately, this is a common occurrence, not just when you start a fitness program but also when you attempt to lose weight. And it can be quite discouraging, since you can go for weeks with no further improvement in your fitness (or with no further weight loss).

You must simply wait it out. Don't slack off on your aerobic program (or stop following your diet). Persistence is the key to making it through a plateau. Eventually, it *will* break. If you know that a plateau probably will occur, you can cope with it better when it does.

Aerobic Points

Dr. Kenneth Cooper has developed a detailed system where you can earn "aerobic points" for your exercise. In his latest book, *The Aerobics Program for Total Well-Being,* Cooper recommends that men obtain at least 35 aerobic points per week and women at least 27.

You can earn 30 points a week, for example, by cycling at 17.5 miles per hour (mph) on a stationary bike for 35 minutes five times a week. Or, if you prefer a faster cadence, try 30 mph for 25 minutes three times a week. If you're interested in Cooper's aerobic points, I suggest that you purchase his latest book.

An Exercise Log

Keeping a log of your indoor cycling program can be extremely helpful. When I first started, I just recorded the date, the miles I'd traveled, how long it took, and any problems I'd had or adjustments I'd made to my bike. Later, after I'd cycled more than 1000 miles indoors, my record keeping became more detailed.

My log is similar to the one shown in Table 5–1. You could either photocopy this log or adopt a similar one. If you make your own, I've found that big sheets of accountant's paper work very nicely and can sit permanently on your reading rack.

With a log, you'll be able to chart your progress. You'll notice changes: Your weight will go down. Your resting pulse will decrease. And you'll need more tension to raise your pulse enough to reach your target zone.

Although it may take a few minutes to fill out the log before and after your workout, it's worth it. You'll be able to look back at where you were two years ago (as I can), and realize how far you've come, and how fit you now are.

YOUR BEGINNING SETUP

Physiologists have discovered that certain bicycling positions and equipment, employed by Olympic level, racing, and touring cyclists, are more efficient than others. Obviously, any you can incorporate into your indoor bicycling will increase your program's efficiency and effectiveness.

Dr. Irwin Faria found that cyclists who grasp the downturned part of "racing" handlebars increase their lung volume by 8.25 percent, compared to when they grasp the upper part of the bars. Apparently, it's easier to expand your chest to breathe deeply when you ride the "drops," thereby increasing the amount of oxygen you consume. Faria concludes a summary of the literature by saying: "To ensure that the cyclist is working toward his greatest

Table 5–1   *Exercise Log*

Day of Week _____

Date _____

Time _____

Starting Mile/Kilometer _____

Ending Mile/Kilometer _____

Total Distance This Workout
   (Miles/Kilometers) _____

Resting Pulse* _____

Location on Map (i.e., "Outside St. Louis") _____

Duration of Workout _____

Intervals (_____minutes at _____
   kpm/min at _____rpm) _____

Average rpm _____

Average Pulse _____

Average Pulse During Intervals _____

Body Weight† _____

Temperature _____

Humidity _____

Heat Rating‡ _____

Calories Used by Workout _____

Adjustments to Bike _____

Motivational "Tricks" _____

Tension Setting _____

Tension During Intervals _____

Average Miles per Hour/Kilometers
   per Hour _____

*Take this before you get out of bed in the morning.
†Take this as soon as you get up in the morning, after visiting the bathroom.
‡Take this reading from Figure 9–1.

potential, the downbar position should be assumed whenever possible. It appears that the body posture adopted by the racing cyclist is crucial for maximal work output, pulmonary ventilation, and energy utilization." So replace your handlebars with downturned bars, and add padding to the bars before you start.

Next, if your stationary bike or ergometer comes with a massive, cumbersome seat, replace it with a sleek racing model. It's the only seat to have for an exercise program.

Then adjust the fore/aft position of your saddle. Although there's not much leeway for this adjustment on stationary bikes or ergometers, this position can be important. Dr. David Smith, writing in *Bicycling* magazine, suggests that you turn the mount of your seat post around so that it rests in *front* of the post rather than behind it. This moves your seat a little farther forward than normal, and aligns your hips and knees better with the pedals. I found this made a tremendous difference in my comfort.

Next, adjust your seat to the correct height. Recent research indicates that saddle height is very important for the proper use of all the leg muscles involved in cycling. Many people place their saddles too low to use their leg muscles adequately. Oddly enough, it's also common for cyclists to raise their seats too *high*. When your seat is too high, it's comfortable for the muscles you use for walking, but you don't learn to use your *bicycling* muscles.

Experiment with various seat heights, but remember that your legs will tire less quickly and help sustain your pace better when your saddle is at the correct height.

Bicycling magazine recommends that you raise your seat to a level where, when your *heels* are on the pedals, you can pedal *backward* without rocking from side to side. If you can't pedal backward at all, lower your seat. If you rock too much on the seat when you back-pedal, raise your seat. If your seat is too high or too low, you'll rock back and forth more than is desirable, which can cause an undue amount of friction and pain.

Dr. Irwin Faria says: "[A] change in seat height changes the range of joint angles that are used to pedal, and this in turn puts the various muscles at different points on their tension-length curves. . . . When the seat height is very low it is likely that the forces tending to dislocate the knee joint are increased considerably. Pain and possible injury far outweigh the benefit of erring on the side of efficiency."

The tilt of your saddle is also important. Keep it level, or maybe tilted slightly upward. Many people tilt their saddle down by mistake, then find that their arms and wrists become very sore after short periods of indoor cycling. Now's the time to add padding to your saddle, too.

Toe clips, accessories that you might think you'd only need outdoors, are invaluable. Dr. Cavanagh's computer work at Penn State indicates that toe clips are vital. He's found that beginners often cycle without toe clips and their feet wander around on the pedals, never producing the correct amount of force in the most efficient position (as they would with toe clips). Without the clips, you also don't make full use of the powerful muscles in the *back* of your thighs. So take time right now to mount your toe clips and adjust their straps.

If you're going to use a reading stand, mount it after you've changed your handlebars and added padding. If you've purchased a heartbeat monitor or bike computer, or plan to listen to tapes or watch television, get that equipment arranged before you start.

Don't forget to place a fan or two directly in front of your bike, so they'll blow onto your face and body. If your bike doesn't have a timer, either mount a clock with a second hand on a wall nearby or wear a watch. If your equipment has a resettable odometer, set it at zero.

It's not necessary to wear a sweat suit, warm-up suit, tights and leotards, or any other form of warm clothing when you cycle indoors. If you're like most indoor bicyclists, you'll warm up very quickly—in fact, you may discover that excess sweat is your problem, not keeping warm! I'd suggest you wear as little as possible.

Under *no* circumstances should you ever wear a rubberized suit when you exercise. They are *extremely* dangerous, and virtually every doctor advises against them. You won't lose more weight when you wear one (contrary to advertising claims), just water that you'll gain back as soon as you take a drink. Rubberized suits can make you so overheated that you faint—or even have a heart attack.

Are you thinking, "If I take all that time, my exercise program will be two hours long every day"? Rest assured that most of this preparation is necessary *only* the first time you ride your indoor equipment. Once all this is set up, you just leave it alone, jump on the bike, and start your warmup.

YOUR BASIC EXERCISE PLAN

Your basic exercise plan will probably look something like this:

- Change clothes. Make any necessary adjustments to the bike.
- Record temperature and humidity. Check to be certain they're not in the "hazard" or "danger" zones of the heat chart (see Figure 9–1).
- Record pertinent information in your log.
- Reset odometer.
- Take the phone off the hook, unplug it, or turn on your answering machine.
- Make sure that your pets and children are in another room and can't unexpectedly sneak in while you're exercising.
- Stretch tight muscles (see Chapter 6).
- Open windows. Turn on fan, or turn off heat (depending on the season).
- Warm up on bike.
- Set timer.
- Do an aerobic session on bike.
- Cool down on bike.
- Stretch any muscles that feel tight (see Chapter 6).
- Do muscular training exercises (see Chapter 6).
- Record information about this workout in your log.
- Take a shower or bath.

Dr. Ed Burke, advisor to the U.S. Olympic Cycling Team, gives some sensible tips about starting your aerobic program: "Don't start out too fast. . . . You need to build your aerobic base by weeks, or possibly months, of steady riding at an accelerated heart rate. These workouts also [will] strengthen your tendons and ligaments so you're better able to try a more strenuous program."

If you're like most beginners, it may seem like forever before you reach your first hundred miles. Then, when your strength and stamina increase, the next few hundred accumulate quickly.

Modify the programs recommended here based on continual monitoring of your heart rate while you exercise. Should your pulse drop lower than your recommended target zone, increase the tension on your bike (or use a more difficult gear on a WLS or rollers). If your pulse goes too high, reduce the tension (or drop to an easier gear).

As long as you keep these simple instructions in mind, you'll *always* work *comfortably* within your recommended target zone.

Week-by-week aerobic schedules are presented for each type of indoor cycling equipment: stationary bikes, ergometers, windload simulators, and rollers.

Start with the very first level, no matter how good you think your fitness is. Then, if your initial workout seems too easy for you, wait until the following day to see if your muscles are sore. If they're not, and if you still feel the workout was too easy, move up a week the next time you ride.

At first, you might find it difficult to bicycle without stopping for 20 minutes. I did. But as you persevere, it becomes much easier. In fact, soon you'll require higher tension at the same cadence to reach the lowest level of your target zone.

You should progress up the chart, even if it's at a slow rate. Some people take two or even three weeks to progress to the next level of difficulty. Use your heart rate as a guide.

Your goal is the maintenance levels on that chart where you'll get enough exercise that your aerobic fitness will be considered "good."

Once you've reached the maintenance level, feel free to experiment. You can exceed those levels if your stamina and leg strength allow. Increase the difficulty of your workout by cycling longer, raising the tension (or cycling in a more difficult gear on a WLS or rollers) or pedaling faster. Just make your changes *gradually,* to reduce any chance of injury to muscles and joints.

THE PROGRAMS

Aerobic Fitness Program: Stationary Bicycle

When you work out on a stationary bike, as I've mentioned before, there's no accurate, reliable measure of the amount of work you're performing. Although each stationary bike recommended in this book has a tension-control device, there's no accurate calibration of the amount of tension produced.

Since you really can't do much more than make general guesses as to whether you're exercising at "low," "low/medium," "medium," "medium/high," or "high" tension levels, you can only figure out how much work you're doing by taking your pulse rate.

The aerobic workouts in Table 5–2 are arranged at progressively more difficult levels, week by week.

To begin your workout, warm up for 5 to 10 minutes at about 15 mph (45 rpm) at no tension or at very light tension. Next, set the tension level so that your pulse reaches the *lower* heart rate figure in your target zone. *Don't* aim for the upper figure immediately, since you'll run a greater risk of injury if you do.

At the beginning, your aerobic phase will last for another 10 minutes at a higher tension. Then cool down for 5 to 10 minutes with no or low tension, as in your warm-up.

Aerobic Fitness Program: Bicycle Ergometer

With a bicycle ergometer, all you need to know to plan your aerobic program is the workload in kilopond-meters per minute (kpm/min) and your cadence (rpm).

The aerobic workouts in Table 5–3 are arranged at progressively more difficult levels, week by week.

If you've purchased a Schwinn ergometer, use the workout plan exactly as it is presented here. If you own a different type of ergometer, compare the kpm/min information with that on your bike.

Note that if your ergometer doesn't give information for various *cadences*, as well as the workload, you can't accurately determine how much work you're doing. Why? Because cycling at 60 rpm, for example, is much less work than cycling at 90 rpm at

Table 5–2　Stationary Bicycle: Aerobic Workouts*

Week	Tension		mph†	rpm	Duration,‡ min	Sessions per Week
1	Low		15	45	10	3
2	Low		17	50	10	3
3	Low/medium		17	50	12	3
	Low/medium	or	24	60	10	3
4	Low/medium		24	60	12	4
	Low/medium	or	27	75	10	4
	Low/medium	or	33	90	8	4
5	Medium		24	60	15	4
	Medium	or	27	75	12	4
	Medium	or	33	90	10	4
6	Medium		24	60	20	4
	Medium	or	27	75	17	4
	Medium	or	33	90	15	4
7	Medium		24	60	25	4
	Medium	or	27	75	22	4
	Medium	or	33	90	20	4
8	Medium/high		24	60	22	4

Table 5–2 *continued*

Week	Tension	mph†	rpm	Duration,‡ min	Sessions per Week
or	Medium/high	27	75	20	4
or	Medium/high	33	90	17	4
9	Medium/high	24	60	25	4
or	Medium/high	27	75	23	4
or	Medium/high	33	90	20	4
Maintenance levels					
	Medium/high	24	60	27	5
or	Medium/high	24	60	32	4
or	Medium/high	27	75	30	4
or	Medium/high	33	90	27	4
or	High	27	75	32	3
or	High	33	90	30	3

*Pedal during warm-up and cool-down at same mph and rpm as rest of that day's workout, but with no or very little tension.

†Using Schwinn's stationary bike as the standard. Rpm and mph relationship may vary on your bike, depending on the size of the flywheel. If you're not sure of the relationship, use mph readings on this chart (or convert them to kph if necessary).

‡Take your pulse once every 5 minutes or so. *Increase* the tension if your pulse is below your recommended target zone. *Decrease* the tension if your pulse is above your recommended target zone.

Table 5–3 Bicycle Ergometer: Aerobic Workouts*†

Week		Workload kpm/min	Schwinn Setting	mph‡	rpm	Duration,‡ min	Sessions per Week
1		150	0.5	24	60	10	3
2		225	0.75	24	60	15	3
3		300	1.0	24	60	15	4
4		375	1.25	24	60	15	4
	or	375	1.25	27	75	15	4
	or	375	1.25	33	90	15	4
5		375	1.25	24	60	20	4
	or	375	1.25	27	75	20	4
	or	375	1.25	33	90	20	4
6		450	1.5	24	60	20	4
	or	450	1.5	27	75	20	4
	or	450	1.5	33	90	20	4
7		525	1.75	24	60	25	4
	or	525	1.75	27	75	25	4
	or	525	1.75	33	90	25	4
8		525	1.75	24	60	30	4
	or	525	1.75	27	75	30	4
	or	525	1.75	33	90	30	4
9		600	2.0	24	60	30	4

Table 5–3 *continued*

Week	Workload kpm/min	Schwinn Setting	mph‡	rpm	Duration,‡ min	Sessions per Week
	or 600	2.0	27	75	30	4
	or 600	2.0	33	90	30	4
Maintenance levels						
	600	2.0	24	60	30	5
	or 600	2.0	27	75	30	5
	or 600	2.0	33	90	30	5
	or 750	2.5	24	60	27	4
	or 750	2.5	27	75	27	4
	or 750	2.5	33	90	27	4
	or 825	2.75	24	60	30	3
	or 825	2.75	27	75	30	3
	or 825	2.75	33	90	30	3

*Pedal during warm-up and cool-down at the same mph and rpm as the rest of that day's workout, but with no or very little workload.

†If you have a Schwinn Air-Dyne, the program shown above is for legs alone *or* arms and legs together. Exercising with arms alone is more strenuous on the Air-Dyne.

‡Using Schwinn ergometers as the standard. Rpm and mph relationship may vary on your bike, depending on the size of the flywheel. If you're not sure of the relationship, use mph readings on this chart (or convert them to kph, if necessary).

§Take your pulse every 5 minutes or so. *Increase* the workload if your pulse is below your recommended target zone. *Decrease* the workload if your pulse is above your recommended target zone.

the same workload. Dials on some ergometers are calibrated so that workload is based on pedal speed.

Schwinn's "Workload Equivalence Scale Conversion Table" (Table 5–4) gives workload equivalents to kpm/min in watts and horsepower. Calorie information is included (which is helpful if you're trying to lose weight), as are comparisons between the difficulty levels of indoor cycling and walking, jogging, and running.

For your first workouts, pedal for 5 to 10 minutes with no

Table 5–4 *Workload Equivalence Scale Conversion Table*,†*

Stationary Exercise	Work Performance			Energy Expenditure‡	Walk/Jog/Run Rate of Exercise (Approx.)	
Load Level Readings	kpm/min	Watts	Horse-power	Calories/min.	Min/mile	mph
0.5	150	24.5	0.033	3	30	2
1.0	300	49.5	0.066	4.5	20	3
2.0	600	100	0.132	7.5	13	4.5
3.0	900	150	0.198	10.5	10	6
4.0	1200	200	0.264	14	8	7.5
5.0	1500	245.3	0.330	17	7	8.5
6.0	1800	300	0.396	20	6	10
7.0	2100	350	0.462	23	5.7	11+

*The table provides work and energy equivalents to the load level readings on Schwinn ergometers. The load level readings given are for standard sea level pressure and 68°F.

†Kpm/min—a measure of work (force) required to move 1 kilogram (2.2 lb.) 1 meter (39+ inches) in 1 min.

Watt—a measure of electric power equal to 6.12 kilopond-meters per minute.

Calorie—a unit of energy based on heat consumption. One calorie equals 200 ml of oxygen consumed. [This chart computed the calorie (heat) expenditure of a 154-lb. person during weight-bearing activity.]

Minute/mile—the time required to cover distance of 1 mile. This is a rate of walk/jog/run intensity to compare with ergometer workload effort requirements.

Mph—a rate of speed used to access the intensity of effort required in weight bearing activities like walk/jog/running.

‡The calorie measure of energy production is affected by body weight/body muscle/fat composition ratio, physical condition, and age. Therefore, this measure will vary from one person to another.

Source: Reprinted with the permission of the Schwinn Bicycle Company, Chicago, Ill.

tension. Try for 24 mph or 60 rpm. Then set the tension at 150 kpm/min. Your heart rate should reach the *lower* level of your target zone during the next 10 minutes (your aerobic exercise). If it doesn't, then try a higher load, such as 225 kpm/min.

Don't aim for the upper level of your recommended pulse range immediately, since, if you do, you run a higher risk of injury.

Cool down for 5 to 10 minutes with no tension.

When I bought my ergometer, I already had put more than 2000 miles on my stationary bike, so I had quite a bit of cycling experience. I started fairly far up on the workout chart, with a load of 525 kpm/min, and progressed from there. (I also find it delightful to know exactly how many calories I've consumed when I ride my ergometer.)

Aerobic Fitness Program: Wind-Load Simulator

Wind-load simulators offer the same accurate, measurable aerobic exercise as ergometers. The advantage of a WLS, as I've mentioned before, is that you can work out on your 10-speed bike.

It's easy to learn to ride a WLS. About the only thing you need to do to get started on your aerobics program (after you've assembled your WLS) is to be sure that all the fittings are tight and your 10-speed bike is totally secure. Then mount and "take off."

The aerobic workouts in Table 5–5 are arranged at progressively more difficult levels, week by week.

To help you understand an aerobics program on a WLS, Racer-Mate has calculated three variables based on the gear and your rpm (Figure 5–2). These are equivalent road speed (mph); horsepower; and calories burned per minute. Racer-Mate also sells a monitor that will give you your mph (or kph) and horsepower.

On a WLS, your warm-up will consist of 5 to 10 minutes of cycling in low, easy gears. You should be "spinning" (as racers describe it), without much tension. After your heart rate rises, and you've just begun to sweat, you're ready to commence your workout.

Your aerobic workout should last another 10 minutes, in a more difficult gear (see Table 5–5). Then, cool down for 5 to 10 minutes in the same easy gear you used for your warm-up.

Table 5–5　Wind-Load Simulator: Aerobic Workouts*

Week	Gear†		rpm	Duration,‡ min	Sessions per Week
1	50		50	10	3
2	50		50	12	3
3	60		60	12	3
4	60		60	15	3
5	70		60	17	4
	70	or	75	12	4
6	70		60	20	4
	70	or	75	17	4
	70	or	90	15	4
7	70		60	25	4
	70	or	75	22	4
	70	or	90	20	4
8	80		60	20	4
	80	or	75	17	4
	80	or	90	15	4
9	80		60	25	4
	80	or	75	22	4

Table 5–5 *continued*

Week	Gear†		rpm	Duration,‡ min	Sessions per Week
9		80	60	25	4
	or	80	75	22	4
	or	80	90	20	4
Maintenance levels					
		90	60	30	5
	or	80	75	30	5
	or	60	90	30	5
	or	100	60	27	4
	or	90	75	27	4
	or	70	90	27	4
	or	100	75	30	3
	or	80	90	30	3

*Pedal during warm-up and cool-down at the same mph and rpm as the rest of that day's workout, but in a gear that offers very little resistance.

†The precise gear will vary depending on the size of your 10-speed bike's chain wheels. Cycle in a gear that's as close to this one as your bike will allow. Determine your gear ratio from Racer-Mate's chart or from the description in the section on aerobic workouts for rollers.

‡Take your pulse every 5 minutes or so. *Increase* the difficulty of your gear if your pulse is below your recommended target zone. *Decrease* the difficulty of your gear if your pulse is above your recommended target zone.

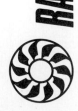

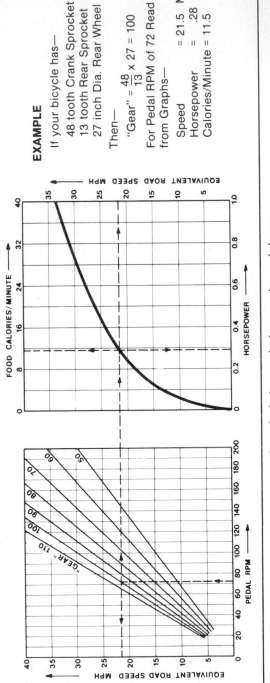

Figure 5–2 Racer-Mate's system for calculating equivalent road speed, horsepower, and calories burned per minute, based on your gearing and pedal rpm. *(Reprinted with the permission of Racer-Mate, Inc., Seattle, WA.)*

When you first begin to work out on a WLS, you'll need to experiment with various gears to see which ones raise your pulse to the *lower* figure of your target zone. *Don't* aim for the upper figure immediately, since, if you do, you'll run a higher risk of injuries.

Mike Kolin, author of Racer-Mate's literature, coaches Seattle's Rainbow Cycling Club. "Our top women riders handle 100 to 110 inch gears (48 × 13 to 52 × 13) for 20 minutes at 70 rpm on the Racer-Mate," he says. "Our top senior men require more load than a *single* Racer-Mate can provide at 70 rpm; therefore, they use the Racer-Mate II with its bottom-mounted turbofan assembly *combined* with the original wind load simulator attached to the seat post. This gives a *double* load." (Emphasis added.) Few readers of this book need a difficulty level that high!

When you're getting on and off your 10-speed bike, be careful not to twist the bike's fork, since you run the risk of bending your frame. In addition, you might want to place a towel across the headset (the top bar of your frame, immediately below your saddle and connecting to your handlebars). Otherwise, your sweat may have a corrosive effect on the paint and metal. You may also want to wipe off and lubricate all moving parts of the WLS every so often.

Be careful when dismounting your WLS so that you don't impale yourself on the upper crossbar. You're considerably higher off the ground than you normally are on a 10-speed bike, so it's easy to forget and jump down. Don't!

Aerobic Fitness Program: Rollers

HOW TO RIDE

You might want to place your rollers in a doorway so that you can steady yourself should you tip over on either side. Unfortunately, I live in a turn-of-the-century house where the door frames are too wide to be of much assistance. But if your home is more modern, you'll have better luck.

Be sure your tires are inflated as high as they'll go without popping. I purchased Schwinn's special reservoir tire pump (see

Appendix A) to inflate my tires, since my portable pump wasn't powerful enough.

Also be sure that the front roller drum is directly under your 10-speed bike's front-wheel axle. Most rollers can be adjusted to your bike's size.

You might want to cover the floor underneath your rollers with a towel, so that your sweat can't harm your carpeting or floor. Additionally, you might cover your bike's stem (the top bar of the frame) with a towel, since roller-riders produce copious quantities of sweat.

Some people use a solid box to mount their rollers; others prefer to purchase steps.

Move anything you wouldn't want to collide with (such as glass mirrors, antique furniture, glass-enclosed bookcases, expensive stereo systems, etc.). Even the best professional roller-riders fall off. One very experienced roller-rider had a tire pop while he was riding and sailed right into a nearby piece of furniture. If something like that can happen to the pros, it can (and probably will) happen to you.

While you are learning to ride rollers, you will definitely require the assistance of a friend. Once you're on the bike, your helper should lightly hold the back of your saddle. Then, start pedaling. Be prepared to feel insecure for the first 15 minutes or so.

Your helper should continue to hold your saddle until you're balancing by yourself. Then the helper can lightly let go, but should remain nearby in case of trouble.

If your helper can't be around, start each ride by leaning against the door frame or a wall. Slowly move away from the wall and begin pedaling. If necessary, put your hand out to steady yourself while you're pedaling.

For the first few workouts, just practice balancing. Try to pedal for a reasonable length of time, perhaps 20 minutes or more. If you can, change gears periodically.

In addition, try to ride with a lower gear and at a higher cadence than you'd use on the road. *Bicycling* magazine says this provides more "gyroscopic stability"—in other words, it's easier to stay on the rollers.

You can also attempt to take your pulse while you ride, although I doubt you'll be able to manage it during your first few tries. In fact, you may find that you never feel secure taking your pulse while riding rollers. In that case, you'll want to invest in a heartbeat monitor or a bike computer that'll tell you your heart rate.

THE AEROBIC WORKOUT

When you work out on rollers, as I've mentioned before, there's no accurate, reliable measure of the amount of work you're performing. You can determine how hard you're working only by regularly taking your pulse, then changing gears if your pulse is below your target zone.

To determine which gears will make your workout more difficult, you must calculate the "gear ratio" of your 10-speed bike. When cyclists discuss "high" and "low" gears, they're referring to the gear ratio in which they're cycling.

When you bicycle outdoors, you use high gears on the flat, low gears on hills. When you cycle indoors, you'll use high gears to keep your pulse up and to ensure that your workout is difficult enough so that you'll reach your target zone.

To calculate your gear ratio, you'll need to count the number of teeth on your bike's front and rear chainwheels. For example, your bike's front chain wheel may have 40 teeth, and the rear 52. The rear cog's teeth might be 14, 17, 20, 24, and 28. After you've counted your bike's teeth, you need to measure your rear wheel's diameter (27 inches is typical). Next, divide the number of chain wheel teeth by the number of rear cog teeth. Multiply by the wheel size.

For example, your gear ratio might look something like this:

	40	52
14	77	100 (highest gear)
17	64	83
20	54	70
24	45	58
28	39 (lowest gear)	50

Type up a small chart that shows your bike's gear ratios, and tape it onto your bike's stem so that you can easily refer to it.

You should warm-up with 5 to 10 minutes of cycling in low, easy gears. You should be only "spinning," as racers describe it. But don't go so slowly that you fall off! After your heart rate rises, and you're only beginning to sweat, you're ready to commence the actual workout.

The aerobic workouts in Table 5–6 are arranged at progressively more difficult levels, week by week. Using the gear ratios in the table as a guide, choose a gear that allows your pulse to reach the *lower* figure for your target zone. Don't aim for the upper figure immediately, since you'll run a greater risk of injury if you do.

At the beginning, your aerobic phase will last for 10 minutes in that gear. Then cool down for 5 or 10 minutes in a low, easy gear—probably the same one you used for your warm-up.

Once you've raised your pulse to the lower level of your recommended range, you should evaluate your first workout.

Some people have difficulty raising their heart rate to the *lowest* level of their target zone, even when they're riding in their most difficult gear. You'll need to experiment to see if you can push your pulse to that level by changing gears.

If not, you'll need to add resistance of some kind. To do this, you could attach an Original Racer-Mate to the back of your wheel. Then use Racer-Mate's guidelines to calculate your work level and follow the guidelines for an aerobic program using a WLS. Or, if you've purchased Kreitler rollers, you'll want to buy the optional blower system that offers all the resistance you could possibly need.

Another thing to try if you can't raise your pulse to your target zone is pedaling at a faster cadence. Unbelievable as it sounds, there are roller-riders who pedal as fast as 200 rpm! I'm not suggesting that you try such an incredible cadence, but you might gradually try to get your rpm rate up around 100, one not uncommon among roller-riders. That cadence requires more work from your heart, even when your gear remains the same.

THE BENEFITS
OF ANAEROBIC TRAINING

Anaerobic training is commonly called *interval training*, and it's used by virtually all endurance athletes. Anaerobic training is an easy way to increase your cycling abilities from one level of aerobic fitness to another.

For example, suppose that you're progressing from week four to week five in the stationary biking program. Instead of suddenly jumping to the higher level, you can add a few anaerobic intervals or *sprints* during the week, cycling perhaps a minute at the higher rate. Then when you reach week five, your heart, muscles, tendons, and ligaments already will have had practice at a higher tension level, and it won't be so difficult to make the transition.

The same benefit of anaerobic intervals holds true when you use an ergometer. If you're aiming for a steady pace of 600 kpm/min, and you've been riding at only 400 kpm/min, you'll find it easier to reach the higher level if you try some 1-minute segments at 600 while you're still cycling primarily at 400.

Intervals also are helpful if you plan to ride outdoors, since they teach your body to cope with hills. Outdoors, the intensity of your cycling varies considerably from the steady-state aerobic pace you maintain indoors.

What you're really doing with anaerobic training is fooling your body into thinking that it's going to exercise at a higher rate, for a longer period, than you actually will. Thus your body gradually learns to adapt to a higher rate of exercise, even though you don't keep up the anaerobic intervals very long.

When you occasionally train at higher levels, your body learns to tolerate intense exercise without quickly shifting into the anaerobic mode. You've raised your *anaerobic threshold* so you're able to cycle at higher intensities without accumulating painful lactic acid.

Your heart's efficiency will also be increased, and it will work at greater intensity without tiring or increasing its *stroke volume* (the amount of blood it pumps per beat).

To create intervals on a stationary bike, WLS, or ergometer, you increase the tension. On rollers without a tension-control device, you create intervals with a more difficult gear.

Table 5–6   Rollers: Aerobic Workouts*

Week	Gear†		rpm‡	Duration,§ min	Sessions per Week
1	39		50	10	3
2	45		50	10	3
3	50		60	12	3
4	50		60	15	3
5	58		60	15	3
	58	or	75	12	3
6	64		60	15	4
	64	or	75	12	4
	64	or	90	10	4
7	70		60	20	4
	70	or	75	17	4
	70	or	90	15	4
8	77		60	20	4
	77	or	75	17	4
	77	or	90	15	4
9	83		60	20	4
	83	or	75	17	4
	83	or	90	15	4

Table 5–6 *continued*

Week	Gear†	rpm‡	Duration,§ min	Sessions per Week
Maintenance levels				
	83	60	27	5
or	83	75	25	5
or	83	90	23	5
or	100	60	27	4
or	100	75	25	4
or	100	90	23	4
or	100	60	32	3
or	100	75	30	3
or	100	90	27	3

*Pedal during warm-up and cool-down at the same mph and rpm as the rest of that day's workout, but in a gear that offers very little resistance.

†The precise gear will vary depending on the size of your 10-speed bike's chain wheels. Cycle in a gear that's as close to this one as your bike will allow.

‡If you find it difficult to count your rpm while riding rollers, you might want to purchase a bike computer that figures it for you (see Appendix A for some recommended brands).

§Take your pulse every 5 minutes or so. *Increase* the difficulty of your gear if your pulse is below your recommended target zone. *Decrease* the difficulty of your gear if your pulse is above your recommended target zone. If you have reached your most difficult gear and your pulse still will not rise into your target zone, you might want to add resistance. (See the discussion in this section.)

Be sure to keep careful track of your heart rate during your interval work. *Never* let your pulse exceed the upper limit of your recommended range. If your heart rate should go higher than that, stop your interval work. *Immediately* return to the aerobic level at which you were previously working. *Don't ever* continue interval training if your heart rate exceeds 85 percent of maximum. It's simply too dangerous.

Intervals should last no longer than 30 seconds to 2 minutes. If you sprint longer, lactic acid will quickly build up and muscle pain will force you to stop. When you return to aerobic cycling after a sprint, your body uses oxygen to dissipate that uncomfortable lactic acid.

An easy way to start is with what Dr. Ed Burke calls *endurance intervals*. After you're about halfway into your typical aerobic workout, continue to pedal at the same cadence, then *slightly* increase the tension. Pedal at that higher intensity for 30 seconds to 2 minutes. Then return to your previous aerobic level.

If you plan a series of these intervals, your pulse *must* return to the level it was at when you started *before* you commence another set. Allow at least 3 minutes between intervals, more if it takes longer for your pulse to come down.

The other type of anaerobic exercise Dr. Burke suggests is *power intervals*. With these, you set the tension considerably higher than your normal aerobic level. Then, at the same cadence as before, ride for 1 to 1½ minutes. Reduce the tension to the aerobic level, then cycle until your heart rate comes down to its earlier reading. Power intervals are considerably more strenuous than endurance intervals and put greater stress on muscles and joints. Don't try them very often.

A final word of warning, however. It's easy to burn out your muscles with an overextended series of intervals. Most researchers recommend that you attempt intervals only once a week or, at the *very* most, twice. They also suggest that you don't consider doing intervals until you've built up *many months* of aerobic fitness.

I suggest that you don't use intervals with any frequency until you reach the maintenance levels recommended in this chapter. Even then, be cautious. Intervals can produce injuries, sprains, and strains. Handle them with care.

Finally, it is not necessary to do intervals at all if you don't want to. You can follow an aerobic program forever, without intervals.

A WORD OF WARNING

One of the most important skills that you should learn, no matter what type of fitness program you participate in, is to listen to your body. Without this ability, you're more likely to suffer from overuse and have pulled or strained muscles.

Pay attention to any unusual aches or pains, and use the "scientific approach" to diagnosing them. If one side of your knee suddenly begins to bother you, but doesn't exactly hurt, see if you've changed your foot's position on the pedals. Are your toe clips loose? Did you forget to tighten the straps before you started cycling? Have you recently increased the tension level, perhaps without building a strong enough fitness base? Any, or all, of these could cause the slight pain in your knee.

Make a few changes in your equipment, and in your cycling program, before you rush to see a doctor or before you stop cycling completely. Many seemingly small irritants are quickly cleared up by this kind of analysis.

It's vital that you pay attention to what your body has to say. Don't ignore the small, irritating, but nonetheless real warning signs of injury-to-come.

Look over these warnings (Table 5–7) and follow the suggestions as to how to cope with any physical problems.

Table 5–7   *Warnings and What to Do About Them*

	Symptom	Cause	Remedy
See a Physician Before Resuming / Stop	1. Abnormal heart action; e.g.: pulse becoming irregular fluttering, jumping, or palpitations in chest or throat sudden burst of rapid heartbeats sudden very slow pulse when a moment before it had been on target (Immediate or delayed)	Extrasystoles (extra heartbeats), dropped heartbeats, or disorders of cardiac rhythm. This may or may not be dangerous and should be checked out by physician	Before resuming exercise program, consult physician who may provide medication to temporarily eliminate the problem, and allow you to safely resume your exercise program, or you may have a completely harmless kind of cardiac rhythm disorder
	2. Pain or pressure in the center of the chest or the arm or throat precipitated by exercise or following exercise (Immediate or delayed)	Possible heart pain	Consult physician before resuming exercise program
	3. Dizziness, lightheadedness, sudden incoordination, confusion, cold sweat, glassy stare, pallor, blueness or fainting (Immediate)	Insufficient blood to the brain	Do not try to cool down. Stop exercise and lie down with feet elevated, or put head down between legs until symptoms pass. Later consult physician before next exercise session
	4. Persistent rapid heart action near the target level even 5–10 minutes after the exercise was stopped (Immediate)	Exercise is probably too vigorous	Keep heart rate at lower end of target zone or below. Increase the vigor of exercise more slowly. If these measures do not control the excessively high recovery heart rate, consult physician

Table 5–7 *continued*

Symptom	Cause	Remedy
5. Flare up of arthritic condition or gout, which usually occurs in hips, knees, ankles, or big toe (weight-bearing joints) (Immediate or delayed)	Trauma to joints which are particularly vulnerable	If you are familiar with how to quiet these flare-ups of your old joint condition, use your usual remedies. Rest up and do not resume your exercise program until the condition subsides. Then resume the exercises at a lower level with protective footwear on softer surfaces, or select other exercises which will put less strain on the impaired joints; e.g. swimming will be better for people with arthritis of the hips since it can be done mostly with the arms. If this is new arthritis, or if there is no response to usual remedies, see physician
6. Nausea or vomiting after exercise (Immediate)	Not enough oxygen to the intestine. You are either exercising too vigorously or cooling down too quickly	Exercise less vigorously and be sure to take a more gradual and longer cooldown
7. Extreme breathlessness lasting more than 10 minutes after stopping exercise. (Immediate)	Exercise is too taxing to your cardiovascular system or lungs	Stay at the lower end of your target range. If symptoms persist, do even less than target level. Be sure that while you are exercising you are not too breathless to talk to a companion

Table 5–7 *continued*

Symptom	Cause	Remedy
8. Prolonged fatigue even 24 hours later (Delayed)	Exercise is too vigorous	Stay at lower end of target range or below. Increase level more gradually
9. Shin splints (pain on the front or sides of lower leg) (Delayed)	Inflammation of the fascia connecting the leg bones, or muscle tears where muscles of the lower leg connect to the bones	Use shoes with thicker soles. Work out on turf, which is easier on your legs
10. Insomnia which was not present prior to the exercise program (Delayed)	Exercise is too vigorous	Stay at lower end of target range or below. Increase intensity of exercise gradually
11. Pain in the calf muscles which occurs on heavy exercise but not at rest (Immediate)	May be due to muscle cramps due to lack of use of these muscles, or exercising on hard surfaces	Use shoes with thicker soles, cool down adequately. Muscle cramps should clear up after a few sessions
	May also be due to poor circulation to the legs (called claudication)	If "muscle cramps" do not subside, circulation is probably faulty. Try another type of exercise; e.g., bicycling instead of jogging in order to use different muscles
12. Side stitch (sticking under the ribs while exercising) (Immediate)	Diaphragm spasm. The diaphragm is the large muscle which separates the chest from the abdomen	Lean forward while sitting, attempting to push the abdominal organs up against the diaphragm
13. Charley horse or muscle-bound feeling (Immediate or delayed)	Muscles are deconditioned and unaccustomed to exercise	Take hot bath and usual headache remedy. Next exercise should be less strenuous

(left margin, vertical:) Can Be Remedied without Medical Consultation

Source: Reprinted with permission from *Beyond Diet . . . Exercise Your Way to Fitness and Heart Health,* courtesy of the Mazola Nutrition/Health Information Service.

6

Complete Your Fitness Program with Stretching and Strength Training

Aerobic fitness, although definitely the most important aspect of your indoor cycling program, is not all the exercise you need. Stretching and strength training are also important to a well-rounded workout.

If you've decided to ride your exercise bike five days a week, you might use that same time period on the other two days for a strength training program. Or add some strength exercises to your cycling days, then rest completely on the other days.

This chapter is not a comprehensive survey of all possible muscular training programs you could follow. Such programs are adequately detailed elsewhere, particularly in books recommended in Appendix B.

I've presumed here that you'll work out at home, without access to Universal gyms or Nautilus equipment.

STRETCHING: SEVEN BASIC EXERCISES

The amount of stretching you need depends on how tight or how flexible your muscles are.

An easy test is to stand with your feet slightly apart, then attempt to touch your toes. Have a friend measure the distance from your fingers to the floor. If you are farther than 9 inches from the floor, your muscles are tight. If you are 5 to 9 inches from the floor, your flexibility is average. And if, like me, you can not only touch your toes but can place your palms flat on the floor, your flexibility is far better than average.

There's another method to measure your flexibility, one that's more precise. Attach a long ruler or tape measure to an uncarpeted floor. Sit down beside the ruler, with your legs extended in front of you. Your legs should be parallel to the ruler, with the 15-inch mark exactly aligned with your heels. Inches 1 to 14 on the ruler should be *toward* your body.

Sit with your legs about 5 inches apart and keep your heels at the 15-inch mark. Also keep the backs of your knees pressed to the floor at all times. Now, bend forward at your waist. Stretch your arms out as far past your toes as you can reach, without allowing the backs of your knees to leave the floor.

Repeat three times. Record the number of inches you reach each time, then average the results. (You might find that it's easier to have a friend take the readings for you.)

Compare your flexibility with these national averages:

Category	Inches
Excellent	22 or more
Good	19–21
Average	14–18
Fair	12–13
Poor	11 or less

Even if your flexibility is normal to loose, don't assume that you don't need to stretch. Remember that any continual exercise such as bicycling or running reduces your flexibility, since the same muscles are used in the same way, day after day. If you don't stretch, you risk pulled muscles that could sideline you for a long time.

Stretch for about 5 minutes both before and after you cycle indoors. In fact, you should stretch whenever you exercise, regardless of whether you're riding your bike or just working out with weights.

Many people make the mistake of bouncing when they stretch. Don't do that. Instead, strive for a gradual, slow stretch to a point from which you know you could stretch farther if necessary. Hold the stretch about 30 seconds (I count "one thousand one," "one thousand two," etc.).

If you feel any pain, gradually ease up on the stretch. Then don't stretch quite so far next time. Give your muscles time to get used to your stretching exercises, but if you have any persistent pain, be sure to see a doctor—preferably someone who specializes in sports medicine.

If your flexibility is low, you probably should do every one of the stretching exercises described in this chapter.

If your flexibility is high, you might be able to skip some exercises. Start, however, by giving them all a try, then eliminate any that are ridiculously easy. But keep watch on your muscles and joints to see if you notice any stiffness when your indoor cycling program becomes more difficult. If this happens, add the stretching exercises designed to loosen that particular area back into your workout.

1. *Achilles tendon stretch:*   Stand next to a wall, press the toes of one foot against the wall while keeping your heel on the floor. Slowly push toward the wall with your knee. You should feel the stretch in your Achilles tendon (at the back of your ankle). Repeat with the other foot. Hold each stretch at least 30 seconds. Longer is desirable, since this tendon often becomes tight from cycling.

2. *Lower back stretch:*   Lie on your back flat on the floor. Pull one knee up to your chest as far as you can while keeping your back and head flat on the floor. Hold for 30 seconds, then repeat with the other leg. This stretches your lower back, rear end, and the hamstrings at the back of your thighs.

3. *Leg stretch:* Sit on the floor with your legs stretched out in front of you. Bend forward from the waist, and try to touch your toes while keeping your legs flat on the floor. Hold for 30 seconds, then return to original position. Repeat. This stretches your legs and lower back.

4. *Hanging stretch:* Stand with feet slightly apart. Bend over from the waist, allowing your arms to hang toward the floor as if you were touching your toes. Hold for 30 seconds, then return to your original position. Repeat. This will stretch your back and the backs of your legs.

5. *Rollover stretch:* Lie flat on your back. Slowly raise your legs up into the air. Then, with your arms and elbows still resting on the floor, roll your legs back over your head. If you're flexible, you should be able to touch the floor *behind* your head with your toes. Hold as long as you can, preferably 30 seconds. Repeat if you can. (This stretch is difficult for many people.) You'll feel the stretch in your lower back, rear end, and in the back of your legs.

6. *Groin stretch:* Sit on the floor. Put the soles of your feet together. Grasp your feet with your hands. Keep your legs flat on the floor. Lean forward toward your toes as far as you can. You're trying to touch your head to your feet. Hold as long as you can, preferably 30 seconds. As the name indicates, this stretch is for the groin area as well as your lower back.

7. *Front-of-leg stretch:* Lie on the floor on your stomach. Keeping your head, chest, and stomach on the floor, reach down with your right hand and pull your right foot up toward your rear end. Hold as long as you can, preferably 30 seconds. Repeat with the other leg. You should feel this stretch in the front of your thigh, the muscles most heavily used by indoor cycling.

STRENGTH TRAINING: TWELVE BASIC EXERCISES

Many bicyclists, from indoor riders to professional racers, experience fatigue in their arms, legs, and back after long bouts of cycling. And what seems "long" is based on your current physical condition. When I first started cycling indoors, 10 minutes was a long time. I now cycle for 40 to 50 minutes, so I suppose that an hour and a half on my ergometer would seem "long" to me.

Many people, in fact, find that their leg or arm muscles get tired *before* they've stressed their cardiovascular system enough to reach their target zone. This was true with me; my heart easily adapted to a heavy cycling regimen, while my thigh muscles still complained.

The solution is strength training. You don't have to start a strength training program right away, although it's a good idea to begin as soon as you're comfortable with your aerobic fitness program—probably after the first six weeks or so.

It's also not necessary to invest in expensive exercise equipment to improve your strength. Nor do you have to join a gym, although many people enjoy the camaraderie of the YMCA or a health club and find that working out with others helps keep them motivated.

If you're a woman, don't worry about becoming muscle-bound. Female hormones ensure that you'll just become firm and taut.

Naturally, there are ways to increase your strength levels on your indoor bicycle. Raise the tension level, which increases the amount of power that you must produce to turn the pedals. If you ride a WLS or rollers, lower gears build strength. You also can, as some professional cyclists do, stand up on the pedals while cycling. *Be careful* when you first try this, however, since many brands of indoor cycling equipment aren't stable when you're standing.

To practice the exercises recommended here, you'll need a pair of ankle weights and a chinning bar. Ankle weights come in 2-, 3-, and 5-pound sizes, and weights with Velcro closures are especially nice. They cost $10 to $20 at any sporting goods store, and you can use them for your arms or legs. The new Heavyhands weight system also might appeal to you. Those hand-held weights are easier to hold than ankle weights, and you can screw on heavier weights as you get stronger.

When you've improved your muscular fitness a little, you might want to buy a weight bench, dumbbells, and barbells. Some of the exercises described here are more beneficial with a weight bench, or are more of a challenge when you use heavier weights.

1. *Toe raises:*   Put a large book on the floor. Stand on its edge so that your toes are on the book while your heels touch the floor. Then raise your heels up as high as you can so that you're balancing on tiptoe on the book. Hold, then come back down. Do five times to start, work up to twenty or more. To increase the difficulty, hold weights in each hand. This exercise will develop and define your calf muscles.

2. *Bicep curls:*   Stand with your feet together. With your arms hanging straight down, hold a weight in each hand, with your palms facing forward. Alternating arms, slowly raise your hands to your shoulders, then slowly return to the starting position. Start with five, work up to twenty or more. This exercise is for the biceps muscles at the front of your upper arm.

3. *Arm swings:*   Sit on the floor, with your legs loosely crossed. With an ankle weight in each hand, extend your arms out in front of your body, palms facing each other. Then, without moving your back, slowly swing both arms simultaneously around to the back of your body, as far as they will go. Your knuckles should be facing each other behind your back. Slowly return to the starting position. Start with five, work up to twenty or more. If you're doing it right, you should feel this in the back of your arms. This exercise is especially beneficial for women who're developing pockets of fat behind their arms.

4. *Bent-knee sit-ups:*   Lie on your back, with your knees *bent* at a 90-degree angle. *Never* do this exercise with your knees straight, since it puts too much strain on your back that way. If necessary, anchor your toes under a heavy couch or another large piece of furniture. Intertwine your fingers behind your head so that your elbows stick out at the sides. Slowly curl up with your head, shoulders, and back, until you're sitting up. Touch your knees with your elbows, or touch one knee with the opposite elbow. Slowly curl back down, and repeat. Start with five (if you can do that many), and increase

to twenty or more. Increase the difficulty by holding a weight behind your head. When done as I've described, you work the abdominal muscles and those on the side of the hips. This exercise helps those "potbelly" problems that men are familiar with.

5. *Crisscrosses:* Lie on your back on the floor. Lift both legs straight up in the air, toes pointed toward the ceiling. Open your legs wide, then bring your right leg across your left. Open again, then cross your left leg with your right. Continue this crisscrossing about ten times. You should feel this exercise in both the inside and outside of your thighs. Work up to twenty or more.

6. *Open-and-closes:* This exercise is similar to the one above. Here, in the same position as in the crisscrosses, you simply open and close your legs without crossing them. You should feel this on the inside of your thighs. Start with ten, increase to twenty or more.

7. *Push-ups:* Lie on your stomach on the floor, with your body fully stretched out and your feet together. Place your hands on the floor next to your head, at approximately shoulder width. Curl your toes under your body. Then push up from that position, supporting your body weight only on your hands and toes. When your arms are fully extended, lower your body back to the floor. Touch your chest only (don't drop all the way down to the floor), then extend your arms fully again. Keep your back straight throughout. Start with one to five repetitions, increase to twenty (if you can). Women will have considerable difficulty with this exercise, since their upper-body strength is usually minimal. They should try to do one, then two, then as many as possible. This exercise strengthens the upper body and shoulders.

8. *Leg raises:* Lie on your stomach on the floor, with your legs outstretched behind you and both feet together. Hold onto the legs of a heavy couch with your hands. Keeping your hips and stomach pressed to the floor throughout, lift your right leg up behind you, as high as possible. Hold for a few seconds, then lower. Repeat with the other leg. Start with five repetitions on each leg, increase to twenty or more. This

exercise is excellent for your rear end, hips and stomach.

9. *Raise-ups:*   Kneel on the floor on your hands and knees. Lift your right leg so your knee is bent, your thigh is parallel with the floor, and your calf is perpendicular to the floor. Your leg will form a sideways L-shape. Point your toes toward the ceiling. Hold this position, without moving, for a count of five.

   Then reach your leg up to the ceiling, maintaining a bent knee. You'll be pulling your thigh back toward your rear end. Come back to the sideways L position. Don't lower your foot below this position, and don't lower it to the floor. Reach up to the ceiling five more times.

   Then lower your right leg and repeat the same procedure with the other leg. Try for five repeats on each leg, work up to twenty. This exercise is excellent for your rear end and the backs of your thighs.

For the next two exercises, you'll need a weight bench, sturdy table, or another flat surface that you can lie on without wobbling.

10. *Arm raises:*   Lie on your back on the bench, holding ankle weights in each hand. Your arms should be extended to your sides, palms facing upward. Raise your arms upward until they're overhead. Keep your elbows locked during the entire movement. Return your arms to your sides. If you find this too easy, you might want to use dumbbells. Start with five and work up to twenty or more. Arm raises work both your chest and shoulder muscles.

11. *Pull-overs:*   Lie on your back on the bench, holding ankle weights in each hand, with your head at the very end of the bench. Place your arms straight overhead, about shoulder width apart. Slowly lower your hands, with elbows fully bent, behind your head as far as possible. Return back to the above-head, extended position. Be careful with this exercise, since your weights will be directly above your face in the overhead extended position. Start with five and work up to twenty or more. This works all the chest muscles.

For the next exercise, you'll need a chinning bar installed in a doorway (preferably a little-used doorway so that no one will run into the bar).

12. *Pull-ups*: Hang from the bar, with your palms, rather than your knuckles, facing your body. Your legs should hang free, not touching the floor. Slowly pull yourself up so that your chin reaches the bar. Don't push with your toes, just use your arms. Lower your body to the starting position, but don't let go of the bar. Repeat. Start with five, work up to twenty or more. This is another exercise that's often difficult for women, since their upper-body strength usually is very low. They should pull up as far as possible, then drop back down. If women keep trying, eventually they'll learn to do one, then more.

For each exercise mentioned, you can increase its difficulty by adding more weight (try two ankle weights instead of one, or dumbbells or barbells with weights), or increasing the number of repetitions.

OTHER EXERCISE

Some people who bicycle indoors supplement their fitness program with other aerobic exercise, thus adding to the variety of their workouts and using muscles not stressed by indoor cycling.

Running is popular with many indoor bike riders, since running develops the hamstrings at the back of the thighs. Running can serve as a complementary activity to bicycling, since cycling primarily works the quads (at the front of the thighs).

Other indoor cyclists work out on rowing machines to develop upper-body strength. Still others enjoy swimming, hiking, racquetball, handball, ice skating, or even dancing, to round out their fitness program. Occasionally, you might enjoy a workout on a "parcours" circuit training course in a nearby park.

The President's Council on Physical Fitness and Sports has rated various activities in terms of their contribution to physical fitness and well being. You may want to use this chart (Table 6–1) as a guide when planning supplemental activities.

Table 6–1   A Quick Scorecard on 14 Sports and Exercises*

	Jogging	Bicycling	Swimming	Skating (Ice or Rolling)	Handball/Squash	Skiing—Nordic	Skiing—Alpine	Basketball	Tennis	Calisthenics	Walking	Golf†	Softball	Bowling
Physical fitness														
Cardiorespiratory endurance (stamina)	21	19	21	18	19	16	19	16	16	10	13	8	6	5
Muscular endurance	20	18	20	17	18	18	17	16	16	13	14	8	8	5
Muscular strength	17	16	14	15	15	15	15	14	14	16	11	9	7	5
Flexibility	9	9	15	13	14	14	13	14	14	19	7	8	9	7
Balance	17	18	12	20	16	21	16	16	16	15	8	8	7	6
General well-being														
Weight control	21	20	15	17	19	15	19	16	16	12	13	6	7	5
Muscle definition	14	15	14	14	11	14	13	13	13	18	11	6	5	5
Digestion	13	12	13	11	13	9	10	12	12	11	11	7	8	7
Sleep	16	15	16	15	12	12	12	11	11	12	14	6	7	6
Total	148	142	140	140	140	134	134	128	126	126	102	66	64	51

Source: Reprinted with the permission of the President's Council on Physical Fitness and Sports.

*Summary of ratings by seven experts. Ratings are on a scale of 0 to 3, thus a rating of 21 indicates maximum benefit (a score of 3 by all seven panelists). Ratings were made on the basis of regular (minimum of four times per week), vigorous (duration of 30 minutes to one hour per session) participation in each activity.

†Ratings for golf are based on the fact that many Americans use a golf cart and/or caddy. If you walk the links, the physical fitness value moves up appreciably.

7

How to Lose Weight with Indoor Bicycling

First, let me give you some background on my own weight "problem." In high school, I weighed 50 pounds more than I do now. I'm 5 feet 8 inches tall and then weighed 180 pounds. Now my weight is stable at 130, and, even more important, my percentage of body fat has gone down to a low of 16 percent. I now slide into a size 7–8 dress, but I vividly remember struggling into an 18–20. And I'm one of only 10 percent of Americans who has lost weight and kept it off. In my case, I've kept it off for more than 10 years.

Now while most of us can lose weight, it's *keeping* the weight off once we return to "normal" eating patterns that is so much more difficult. It requires a genuine, and, for most people, life-long commitment. Bicycling indoors will help you take it off *and* keep it off.

OVERWEIGHT AND OVER-FAT

Before we go on, however, it's necessary to clear up a common misconception: "Overweight" and "over-fat" are not the same thing. You *must* understand the difference before you try to lose weight.

Overweight simply means that you weigh more than the average American of your sex and height. This can be determined by comparing your weight to insurance industry tables (Table 7–1). To determine your frame size, use Metropolitan Life's guidelines (Table 7–2).

These two tables can help you determine whether you're "overweight" by insurance industry standards (which many doctors believe are too high since they represent averages, not "ideals"). What the tables won't tell you is whether or not you're *over-fat*.

You actually can be overweight by the tables, yet have a very small percentage of fat on your body. Many professional football players, for example, are overweight, yet they have only 5 percent fat on their bodies.[1]

The classic case of someone who's over-fat is the pro ballplayer who, 10 years after he retired, still weighs 225 pounds. Unfortunately, he stopped exercising, so the percentage of body fat he's now carrying is close to 30 percent. He constantly hears jokes about how his broad chest slipped down to his stomach.

The opposite case also applies. You can weigh considerably *less* than the values shown in the insurance tables, yet be over-fat. An example might be a woman who's never exercised much, yet has kept her weight constant at 115 pounds. Unfortunately, as she ages, rolls of fat begin appearing here and there, and her legs and upper arms look flabby. Yet her weight is *below* that suggested by the tables. Still, she's over-fat.

Two women of the same height can both weigh 120, yet wear two different dress sizes. One, who rides her bicycle ergometer 30 minutes a day and has little body fat, takes a size 7–8. The other, who follows no regular exercise program and has a sedentary office job, takes an 11–12.

[1]Dr. Jean Mayer, internationally recognized nutritionist and president of Tufts University, believes athletes often are mistakenly described as overweight because muscle forms such a large proportion of their total body weight.

Table 7–1 *1983 Metropolitan Height and Weight Tables**

Men				
Height		Frame Size		
Feet	Inches	Small	Medium	Large
5	2	128–134	131–141	138–150
5	3	130–136	133–143	140–153
5	4	132–138	135–145	142–156
5	5	134–140	137–148	144–160
5	6	136–142	139–151	146–164
5	7	138–145	142–154	149–168
5	8	140–148	145–157	152–172
5	9	142–151	148–160	155–176
5	10	144–154	151–163	158–180
5	11	146–157	154–166	161–184
6	0	149–160	157–170	164–188
6	1	152–164	160–174	168–192
6	2	155–168	164–178	172–197
6	3	158–172	167–182	176–202
6	4	162–176	171–187	181–207
Women				
Height		Frame Size		
Feet	Inches	Small	Medium	Large
4	10	102–111	109–121	118–131
4	11	103–113	111–123	120–134
5	0	104–115	113–126	122–137
5	1	106–118	115–129	125–140
5	2	108–121	118–132	128–143
5	3	111–124	121–135	131–147
5	4	114–127	124–138	134–151
5	5	117–130	127–141	137–155
5	6	120–133	130–144	140–159
5	7	123–136	133–147	143–163
5	8	126–139	136–150	146–167
5	9	129–142	139–153	149–170
5	10	132–145	142–156	152–173
5	11	135–148	145–159	155–176
6	0	138–151	148–162	158–179

Source: Data from 1979 Build Study, Society of Actuaries and Association of Life Insurance Medical Directors of America, 1980.

*Weights at ages 25–59 based on lowest mortality. Weight in pounds according to frame (in indoor clothing weighing 5 pounds for men and 3 pounds for women; shoes with 1-inch heels.)

Copyright 1983 Metropolitan Life Insurance Company; reprinted courtesy of the Metropolitan Life Insurance Company.

Table 7–2   *Approximation of Frame Size*

To make an approximation of your frame size . . .	Height in 1-in. heels	Elbow Breadth (in.)
	Men	
	5'2"–5'3"	2½–2⅞
	5'4"–5'7"	2⅝–2⅞
	5'8"–5'11"	2¾–3"
	6'0"–6'3"	2¾–3⅛
	6'4"	2⅞–3¼
	Women	
	4'10"–4'11"	2¼–2½
	5'0"–5'3"	2¼–2½
	5'4"–5'7"	2⅜–2⅝
	5'8"–5'11"	2⅜–2⅝
	6'0"	2½–2¾

Extend your arm and bend the forearm upward at a 90-degree angle. Keep fingers straight and turn the inside of your wrist toward your body. If you have a caliper, use it to measure the space between the two prominent bones on *either side* of your elbow. Without a caliper, place thumb and index finger of your other hand on these two bones. Measure the space between your fingers against a ruler or tape measure. Compare it with these tables that list elbow measurements for *medium-framed* men and women. Measurements lower than those listed indicate you have a small frame. Higher measurements indicate a large frame.

Source: Reprinted courtesy of the Metropolitan Life Insurance Company.

Thus, you can be any of the following: overweight and not over-fat; over-fat and not overweight; overweight as well as over-fat (this seems to be typical in America); or, the ideal, neither overweight nor over-fat.

While the insurance tables will tell you whether or not you're overweight, determining whether you're over-fat is a little more complicated.

HOW MUCH FAT DO YOU HAVE?

One way to judge your fat level is the *jiggle test* recommended by Dr. Kenneth Cooper. It's easy to do—you just stand nude in front of a full-length mirror, then jump lightly up and down. Anything that jiggles is fat. Anything that doesn't is muscle.

Another informal way is the *pinch test*. Simply pinch your fat at various locations on the body. Wherever you pinch more than one inch of fat, you're over-fat. Women usually find they pinch too much on the front and back of their thighs, on the backs of their arms, and on their abdomens and buttocks. Men find more fat on the abdomen and at the waistline. However, the hormone estrogen ensures that the average woman will *always* have more fat than the average man.

Average body fat for women is 22 to 25 percent. Average values for men are 12 to 15 percent. Dr. I. Faria recommends that women bike racers strive for fat levels of 8 to 13 percent, while men racers get down to 5 to 8 percent, but those levels may be too low for you.

Now there's another method to estimate your body fat. You use what's known as the Figure Finder Tape Measure. The tape comes with a "tensioning device" that ensures consistent, repeatable measurements. This innovative device guarantees that you can't pull the tape tighter instead of losing inches!

Novel Products (the company that also makes the inexpensive skin caliper discussed below) says their tape measure has a guaranteed accuracy level of 3/32 inch on its 60-inch length, as well as a consistent and repeatable tension of 4 ounces. A booklet tells you how to take twelve body measurements, and tables (such as Figure 7–1) explain how men estimate their body fat from their waist measurement. Women can figure their body fat from their hip measurements.

The tape costs only $4.99. It's a worthwhile investment for anyone who's losing weight or who just wants to maintain body fat at a low level.

Finally, there are two scientific methods that can be used to measure your fat. For the first, you need to visit a sports fitness center, university physical education department, or rehabilitation center where they do underwater weighing. You are weighed both in and out of the pool. The difference between the two figures indicates what your "lean body weight" is—your weight excluding fat deposits.

The second method to measure your body fat is by using a skinfold caliper, an instrument designed to show very small differences in fat levels on various locations of your body (see Figure 7–2). Pressure used in measuring fat is constant, since it's built into the caliper. No mechanical variation affects your readings.

Typically, measurements are made at six locations, including your chest, arm, back, hip, abdomen, and thigh (see Figure 7–3). You'll need a friend to help you do this.

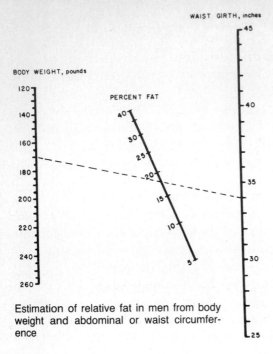

Estimation of relative fat in men from body weight and abdominal or waist circumference

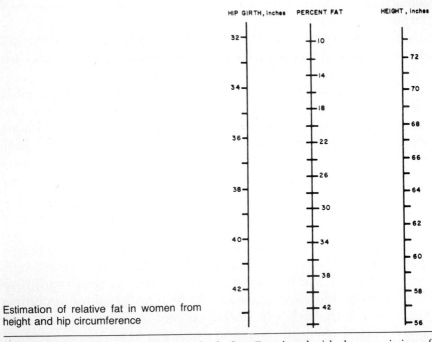

Estimation of relative fat in women from height and hip circumference

Figure 7–1 Estimation of relative body fat. (Reprinted with the permission of Dr. Jack H. Wilmore from *The Wilmore Fitness Program*.)

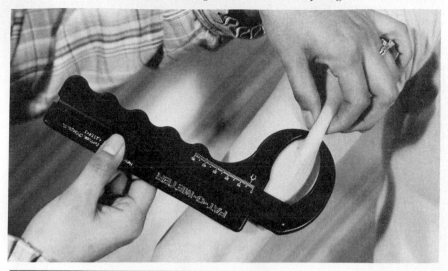

Figure 7–2   The $9.95 Fat-O-Meter skinfold caliper. (Courtesy of Novel Products, Inc., Addison, IL.)

Your *chest* skinfold measurement should be taken at a location on the front of your chest that's below your shoulder, above your breast, and near your arm. Your *arm* measurement should be taken at the back of your arm, above the elbow. Measure your *back's* fat at a location just below the lower part of your shoulder blade.

Hip measurements should be taken at the side of your body, just below the waist. Measure your *abdomen's* fat at the center of your waistline, approximately next to your navel. *Thigh* measurements should be taken at the front of your thigh, about midway between your knee and the top of your thigh.

When you repeat these skinfold measurements, be sure that you measure on the same side of your body—that is, if you take all measures on your right side, be sure to use the right side the next time you take your skinfolds.

When using a skinfold caliper, your helper (who will take the measurements) must be careful to "pick up" your skin in the same manner every time. Standard procedure is to use the thumb and forefinger of your left hand. Hold them just far enough apart so that you can pick up a fold of skin from the tissue below. Don't grasp firmly, just "pluck up" skin. Don't pull up the larger tissues

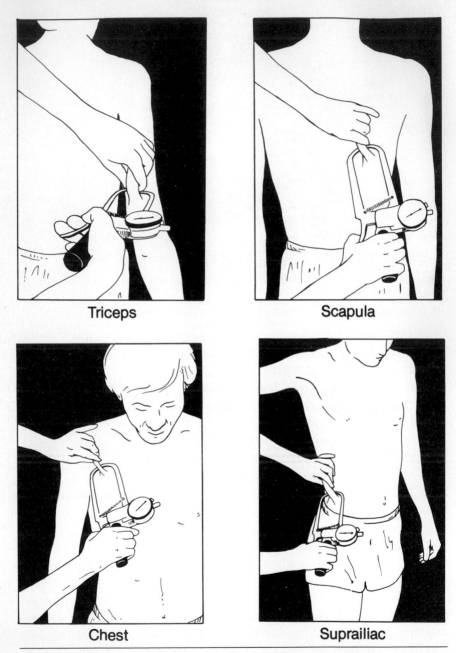

Triceps

Scapula

Chest

Suprailiac

Figure 7-3 How to measure body fat at six locations. (Reprinted with the permission of Dr. Jack H. Wilmore from *The Wilmore Fitness Program*.)

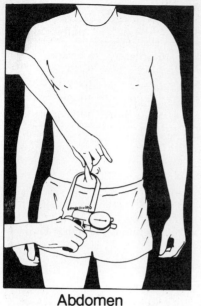

Abdomen

Thigh

Figure 7–3 *Continued*

that lie under your skin. The calipers should be applied only *below* the fingers, so the pressure on the measurement site is only that from the calipers.

Compare your skinfold measurements with the standards listed by Theodore Berland in his excellent *Fitness Fact Book* (Table 7–3).

For anyone with a weight problem, I consider owning a skinfold caliper equally—if not more—important than a bathroom scale. For a long time, however, the only calipers available cost about $200, a price that was prohibitive for most dieters.

Recently, an innovative Chicago company, Novel Products, patented a $9.95 skinfold caliper (see Figure 7–2). Please don't assume that because this caliper is cheap, it's therefore inferior. To the contrary. Extensive research at the University of Wisconsin has found the $9.95 Fat-O-Meter to be as accurate and reliable as the $200 models. And the spring is designed to take over 1 million readings without any loss of tension. I can't recommend the Fat-O-Meter too highly.

Table 7–3 *Skinfold Chart (measured in millimeters)**

	Chest	Arm	Back	Hip	Abdomen	Thigh
Excellent	6 or less	5 or less	6 or less	6 or less	8 or less	6 or less
Good	7–12	6–7	7–12	7–12	9–15	7–10
Average	13–21	8–11	13–21	13–22	16–29	11–18
Fair	22–26	12–15	22–27	23–30	30–39	19–24
Poor	27 or more	16 or more	28 or more	31 or more	40 or more	25 or more

*Measurements are taken as shown in Figure 7–3:
Chest—chest drawing.
Arm—triceps drawing.
Back—scapula drawing.
Hip—suprailiac drawing.
Abdomen—abdomen drawing.
Thigh—thigh drawing.
Source: Reprinted from *The Fitness Fact Book* with the permission of author Theodore Berland

WHAT'S YOUR BMR?

Before you can commence a weight-loss program, you'll need to calculate your *basal metabolic rate* (BMR). The BMR is the amount of calories your body uses in everyday activities, with no added exercise. The easiest way to figure your BMR is to use the following table. If in doubt, estimate *low*.

Activity Level	To Obtain BMR, Multiply Your Weight by:
Sedentary	13
Moderately active	15
Active for most of the day	20

Most Americans are sedentary. Office workers, most housewives, retail workers, and close to 80 percent of our population fit into the sedentary category. You probably do, too, unless you get some continual exercise during the day.

If you walk to work, swim at lunch, move boxes around part of the day, walk on the job, ride your outdoor bike and do calisthenics, or otherwise engage in an hour's worth of exercise every day, you're probably moderately active.

Finally, you fit into the category "active most of the day" only if you exercise more than two to three hours a day, have a job where you exercise virtually all day long, ride a bike or walk long distances to work, work as a manual laborer, or otherwise exercise for long hours every day. Very few Americans belong in this category.

If you weigh 140 and are moderately active, for example, your BMR is 140×15, or 2100 calories per day. By consulting the weight chart, you've decided you should reduce to 125 pounds. Multiply 125 by 15 to get 1875 calories per day—the amount you'll be able to eat without gaining once you reach your ideal weight. Since your BMR goes down when you lose weight, you must eat *less* than you did at a higher weight to maintain your new weight permanently.

WHY SHOULD YOU EXERCISE
WHEN YOU'RE TRYING TO DIET?

Isn't dieting bad enough? That's a natural, but incorrect, reaction. Actually, you lose weight more quickly when you combine diet with exercise. You'll also lose fat more quickly when you add exercise to your diet. Research studies also indicate that when you exercise while you're dieting, you lose fat, *not* water or protein from vital body organs or muscle tissue as you can if you don't exercise.

You'll also feel better when you exercise and diet. You'll have more energy to confront the day cheerfully, and you'll sleep better. Your brain will receive more oxygen. In fact, all the positive benefits of exercise mentioned in Chapter 2 apply when you're dieting.

A regular, sustained, consistent exercise program will not only reduce the amount of fat present in your body, but can also increase your BMR. If you start cycling indoors for at least a half-hour a day, your BMR probably will increase. Thus, your new exercise not only uses up calories, but also "turns up" your body's metabolism. In fact, some studies indicate that exercise can increase BMR for as long as 24 hours after you finish.

Also, don't forget the difference in the amount of calories you can eat based on your activity level. A sedentary 125-pound woman only uses 1625 calories per day. If, however, the same woman incorporates a half-hour or more of indoor bicycling per day at 10 calories per minute, and some calisthenics, her BMR probably will increase to the moderately active level of 1875 calories. In addition, she has used 300 calories cycling.

Probably the most important benefit of exercise while dieting, however, is that your muscles firm up while you lose weight, so there's no flabbiness or stretch marks that linger as a result of your diet.

Perhaps you've never seen anyone who's lost prodigious quantities of weight without exercising. I have. An acquaintance once followed a balanced diet (recommended by a major group weight-loss program) for almost a year, and lost 150 pounds. However, she did not exercise during that period, and, as a result, her skin literally "hung" on her. Her upper arms had two huge "flaps" on them, 6 or 7 inches long. And the backs of her thighs had the same awful "flaps" of skin, but much larger, perhaps 10 to 12 inches. She was considering plastic surgery to remove that excess skin. Yet if she had exercised, she'd have had no need for an operation. She's an intelligent woman, but was simply ignorant of the virtues of exercise and the irreparable damage that can be done if you strenuously diet without it.

Dr. Jean Mayer is world famous for his studies on lack of exercise and its inexorable companion, obesity. Human beings, like animals, gain weight when their activity is severely restricted. In fact, Dr. Mayer found one group of more than 200 adults who had become overweight as a *direct* result of a sudden decrease in their activity.

Mayer's most famous study was conducted in India; it compared caloric intakes with body weights of workers in various occupations. He grouped workers according to the amount of exercise they received each day. Mayer's results are striking: Below a certain minimal level of exercise, people apparently eat *more* calories than they need, so they weigh too much. At a reasonable level of exercise, they eat a moderate amount of food, and their weight is normal. When their job requires a strenuous level of exercise, their calorie consumption goes up. Their weight, however, does *not*.

In another study, Mayer found that obese adolescent girls in Massachusetts ate *less*, not more, than their friends of normal weight. But the obese girls spent two-thirds less time in daily activities that involved any exercise. Unfortunately, the heavy girls thought they ate *more* than their slim friends, and didn't realize they really were exercising less, not eating more.

Dr. I. Faria, author of *Cycling Physiology for the Serious Cyclist*, says: "Changes in body composition associated with chronic exercise programs include a slight decrease in total body weight, a moderate decrease in body fat, and a moderate increase in lean body weight." In fact, he states: "If an individual undergoes a strenuous conditioning program, body weight may increase despite a decrease in body fat. The added muscle mass being more dense than fat is responsible for such an increase in weight. At the same time, certain body dimensions may decrease even though the body weight remains the same or even increases slightly. Again, this can be explained by the fact that muscle tissue had replaced fat tissue."

HOW TO LOSE WEIGHT (AND FAT)

Once you find your ideal weight based on the insurance industry tables, compare your skinfold measurements with those presented here, and calculate your BMR, you're ready to embark on a program to lose weight *and* fat.

Let's return to our example of a woman who's begun an indoor bicycling program that uses 300 calories a day. Her BMR is now a moderately active 1875, to which she adds 300 calories, for a daily total of 2175 calories that's required to sustain her weight.

Suppose that she normally eats 2100 calories per day. If she doesn't exercise, she'll eat approximately 475 calories a day too many. At that rate, she'd gain a pound every week or so. (A pound of fat is equivalent to 3500 calories.)

However, with an indoor cycling program at 2100 calories, she'll maintain her weight. Actually, she'd *lose* very slowly, since her exercise is using up an extra 75 calories a day. At that rate (a slow and discouraging weight loss for most people), she'd lose a pound about every 46 days.

But if she starts a diet at the same time she begins her exercise program, she'll lose weight more quickly *and* she'll lose fat and inches at the same time. If she chooses a 1500-calorie a day diet (which most women don't consider particularly stringent) and bicycles indoors every day, her total daily caloric deficit would be $2175 - 1500 = 675$ calories. At that rate, she'll lose a pound about every five days. Since most nutritionists and doctors recommend that you lose no more than 1 or 2 pounds a week, this would be just about right.

Naturally, our hypothetical woman could lose more weight by reducing her caloric intake even more, *or* by increasing her exercise. She could drop her calories down to 1200 per day (the lowest a woman should go to ensure adequate intake of protein, vitamins, and minerals). At that rate, her deficit would be $2175 - 1200 = 975$ calories, and she'll lose a pound every $3\frac{1}{2}$ days, or approximately 2 pounds a week. If she keeps losing at that rate, she'll lose 10 pounds in 5 weeks, 20 pounds in 10 weeks, or 30 pounds in 15 weeks. And she stands a good chance of keeping the weight and fat off—especially if she continues her exercise program.

Remember that you'll need to recalculate these figures every time you lose 10 pounds or so.

The American College of Sports Medicine recently made a series of recommendations as to the best way to lose weight and fat. Based on an extensive review of weight-loss literature, they suggest you:

• Don't fast. Don't attempt quick-weight-loss fad diets.

• To lose fat, not necessary nutrients, reduce your caloric intake by no more than 500 to 1000 calories per day.

• Don't lose more than 2 pounds per week.

• Eat at least 1200 calories per day, *never* less.

• Exercise at least three days per week, for at least 20 minutes, at an intensity of at least 60 percent of your maximum heart rate. Use at least 300 calories per session. (If you exercise four times a week, you should use at least 200 calories per 20-minute session to lose body fat.)

• Plan to keep up an exercise program, combined with careful eating, forever.

• Try behavior-modification techniques if you have trouble sticking to a diet.

The College suggests that if you attempt to lose weight quickly (perhaps by the latest "orange rinds and mustard" diet), you only succeed in upsetting numerous metabolic balances essential for good health. And you'll probably lose water, minerals, and body tissues other than fat, adding to your subjective feelings of ill health while you diet.

If you'd like more details on sensible, well-balanced weight-loss diets, I'd suggest you read Dr. Jean Mayer's excellent books *Overweight* and *A Diet for Living*, or obtain a copy of *Consumer Guide* magazine's fine annual review, *Rating the Diets*. Author Theodore Berland describes virtually every diet presently popular in the United States, no matter how oddball the diet may be. He gives four-star ratings to a number of diets that follow the U.S. Senate's Dietary Goals and are well-balanced and safe. I'm sure you'll find one to your liking in the four-star group.

Personally, I've followed the Pritikin/Live Longer Now diet for years. It's high in carbohydrates and whole grains, and low in salt, sugar, and fats. I feel terrific on this diet.

Dr. David L. Smith reminds you to expect a 3- to 5-pound weight regain when you complete your diet, which is the water you lost at the beginning of your diet.

Women should be sure that their reducing diet contributes the minimum daily requirement of iron. Without enough iron, your body's ability to carry oxygen to your cells is considerably reduced. This lack of oxygen, in turn, can lower your body's ability to handle an aerobic fitness program.

Some research done with subjects who rode bicycle ergometers indicates that eating more frequent meals can improve your exercise ability. Other studies indicate that four or five small meals (or three meals with one or two snacks) fend off hunger pangs better.

If you're pregnant, or have any physical problems that might affect whether you should diet, check with your doctor. Remember that you can lose weight (although more slowly) by exercise alone, without dieting.

INDOOR CYCLING
AND WEIGHT LOSS

Once you've chosen a reducing diet and calculated how many calories you consume per day, you're ready to figure out how many calories you use by indoor bicycling.

Indoor cycling is rather unique, when compared with other exercises, in terms of calories used. Since your body is supported by an indoor bicycle, there is *no* difference in calories used based on your weight. This is different from activities such as walking or running, where if you weigh more than your friend you use more calories, since you move more weight with every step. With indoor cycling, however, you use the same number of calories for the same amount of work as your friend does.

This fact actually can be an advantage for those who are extremely overweight. Since indoor cycling does not require you to move around, or pound excess weight against hard asphalt, many heavy people find it an easy aerobic fitness program to follow.

One of the biggest advantages of an indoor cycling program or an ergometer or WLS is their ability to measure precisely the calories you've consumed. You won't have to figure out how many miles you've run through your neighborhood or how far that evening walk around the park was. All you have to do is look at the workload monitor or Racer-Mate's chart, and you'll immediately know how many calories you've used.

Of course, the longer or harder you cycle indoors, the more calories you use. If you cycle at a rate that uses 8 calories per minute and ride 20 minutes, you use 160 calories. If you cycle for 30 minutes, it's 240 calories, and at 40 minutes, you consume 320 calories. Or if you increase the amount of difficulty of your workout so that you're using 10 calories a minute, at 20 minutes you use 200 calories; at 30 minutes, 300 calories; and at 40 minutes, 400 calories.

Caloric differences occur in indoor cycling only by virtue of the amount of *work* you do. Therefore, even though your heart rate increases, perhaps on a day that's hot and humid, that unfortunately doesn't indicate that you're using more calories. I wish it did.

If you own an ergometer, your bike might come with a stick-on label that gives calorie use for various workloads, or your instruction book might provide that information. If not, you can use Table 5–4 to determine how many calories you've used, since virtually every ergometer measures work either in kilopond-meters per minute (kpm/min) or watts. That table's calorie figures apply to all ergometers. Racer-Mate's chart (Figure 5–2) gives calorie consumption figures for wind-load simulators.

If you have a stationary bike, you might ride an ergometer at a gym or a friend's to get an idea of what workload you've been cycling at. Then, using an educated guess, you can figure out approximately how much work you're doing. I realize this isn't the best solution, but to be precise you must purchase an ergometer or WLS.

If you plan to cycle outdoors, either to supplement your indoor fitness program or on the weekends, you can use the calorie figures from Figure 7–4. When you cycle outdoors, your body weight *does* affect the calories you use per hour. The heavier you are, the more energy you use to propel the bike on the flats and on the hills. And the heavier you are, the more slowly you climb hills. But while you're puffing up those hills, remember that even though you may be slower than your skinny friend, you're also using *more* calories per mile, and you'll steadily lose weight if you keep cycling.

Oddly enough, the opposite effect occurs when you're going downhill. If you're overweight, you'll often pass your friend on the downhills, because gravity is attracted to your higher weight.

If you're like me—with a life-long tendency to gain weight easily—take heart. You *can* lose weight to your recommended level, and you *can* keep it off. Although there is no sure-fire, quick-and-easy way to lose weight, a slow, steady pace *does work*, and you'll be far more likely to banish those extra pounds forever if you don't try "quickie" methods.

When you combine reasonable exercise program (such as the

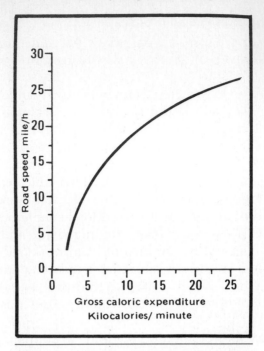

Figure 7–4   Gross caloric expenditure for a cyclist who weighs 170 lb. (Reprinted with the permission of editor Barbara George from *Inside the Cyclist*, published by *Velo-news*, Brattleboro, VT, 1982.)

one I recommend here) with sensible eating, you'll be able to maintain your newfound weight virtually forever.

But never forget that exercise plays a vital, irreplaceable role, both in the original loss of weight *and* fat and in long-term maintenance of your goal weight.

I genuinely hope that you're as successful as I've been.

8

Motivational Tips

Luckily, I've never been bored during the three years I've been cycling indoors. In fact, I hadn't realized that other people consider indoor cycling a "boring" form of exercise until I started doing research for this book.

But it *doesn't* have to be boring.

You should know, however, that realistically the first six weeks of your program will be the most difficult. Until your exercise program becomes as much of a daily habit as brushing your teeth (which takes about six weeks), you'll need to "trick" yourself into cycling.

But rest assured that after that time, indoor cycling will be a habit, and you'll feel so strong, healthy, energetic, and fit from your program that you won't even consider discontinuing it.

Now that I've been cycling for almost three years, it's a joy to get up and ride my bike. I know how good I feel throughout the day when I bike in the morning. And that knowledge propels me up and onto my bike.

One ploy I've used to keep myself motivated is to place my bike where I can't possibly miss it. I keep my ergometer at the foot of my bed, so I fall over it when I get up in the morning. Every morning, without fail, I force myself to choose whether to cycle indoors or not. And practically every morning, I do.

So get that bike out in the open, where you force yourself to walk around it or trip over it. It's fine if you decide later that you'd rather ride your bike in the garage, basement, or attic. Once your first six weeks are up, you can put your bike wherever you like.

I also make daily appointments to bike in my datebook. I write "Bike" at the beginning of the day. Since I'm in the habit of checking my datebook before I go to bed and first thing in the morning, I always see this reminder. When I finish cycling, I check off that entry just as I do my business appointments.

My favorite game is tracing my imaginary progress across the United States on a map. I'm a blue pushpin. Every time I pass 25 miles, I move the pin along.

Somehow your accumulated mileage means more when you "see" it in real distances. It makes no difference whether you cycle across the United States, or Canada, or Australia, or around the world (even across the Atlantic, if you'd like). You can have a lot of fun with this game. First, it's silly. After all, who ever heard of bicycling across the United States without leaving your bedroom? Your friends will think you're crazy . . . then they'll soon get in the spirit of the joke. Sometimes when conversation lags, I'll say, "I'm in Flagstaff now," or "I rode into Davenport this morning." My friends do a double-take, then chuckle when they realize what I'm talking about. It's also a marvelous filler at parties when conversation slows down. Try tossing off, "I bicycled into El Salvador this morning," and watch the heads turn!

A friend who regularly rides an exercise bike took my idea a step further. He writes to the Chamber of Commerce of towns that he'll soon "reach" and accumulates travel brochures from them. Then he keeps the brochures on his reading stand and leafs through them while he pedals. He says this has "made my trips come alive," and he's now planning a bicycle trip (outdoors, this time) that will take him to many of the places he's already "visited."

In addition to traveling across the United States, you will probably simply enjoy accumulating mileage. When my odometer turned over for my first thousand miles, I started cheering.

You can even set monthly or annual mileage goals for yourself. Try something like "I want to cycle between New York and Boston this month," or "I want to bike two hundred miles this month." Or challenge yourself with a cross-country trip within one year. Keep your goals reasonable, however—within your capabilities. If you're brand-new at indoor cycling, don't expect to cross the United States this year. But in two years. . . .

Write down your goals, preferably in your log or on a sign next to your map. Psychological studies indicate that when you write something down, you'll continue to do it in the future, but if you don't write it down, you won't. When you keep a log, you play on this natural tendency, and you'll learn to set goals and compare your steady progress.

I've also scheduled mini-celebrations for myself when I reach my goals, such as a thousand miles or arriving in New York from Los Angeles. I do something special, such as go to the theater or to a movie as a reward. And, of course, I tell my friends (and gloat a little). And I just feel proud of myself for achieving such a major goal.

Another way to have fun on your indoor bicycle is to read while you exercise. This is especially helpful when you are starting out, since it helps you stick to your program. It certainly helped me. I simply attached a reading stand to my handlebars. During my first 300 miles or so, I read a number of interesting books, and sometimes forgot I was exercising when I got engrossed in my reading. However, for some inexplicable reason I couldn't concentrate on fiction when I cycled, so I stuck to nonfiction.

I continued my reading until my fitness improved and I could cycle at a higher cadence. When I exceeded 30 mph, however, I found I couldn't read. So I converted my reading stand to a daily log holder, and now read only during my warm-up and cool-down.

You might find you enjoy reading a newsmagazine you otherwise never have time for, or the morning paper, or a business journal. I prefer a book, however, so that I don't reach the end before my workout's done.

Or, if you like to read but find you can't concentrate while riding your indoor bike, try listening to books on cassette tapes.

You should also try to cycle at a pedal speed of over 70 rpm. Virtually the only time I've found myself getting bored while cycling was when I was going only 60 rpm while using a high tension level. When I could stand the boredom no longer, I went back to my normal 90 rpm. Immediately my boredom disappeared. I can't explain this, and have found no research studies confirming my perceptions. But for me (and for many people) a low cadence produces instant, intense boredom, while a high cadence does not. And, as I've mentioned before, a higher cadence is *much* kinder on your knees, ankles, and feet.

Adding variety to your workout keeps you motivated. I've found that when I cycle intervals, the time goes very quickly. I ride normally for 4 minutes, then do a 1-minute interval. Then I ride normally for 4 more minutes, and repeat the interval.

Many people like to watch television while they ride their indoor bikes. In fact, you can incorporate bike riding with your favorite daily programs. Or if you're not home for your favorite show, just program your videotape machine to record it, then ride your bike to the show later. Or you could film your own home movies or videotapes, perhaps of beautiful nearby roads or cycling trails, and watch them while you cycle.

It makes no difference whether you cycle to the noon or evening news, a feature-length movie, your own videotapes, a soap opera, or a game show. What you're doing is conditioning yourself to ride your exercise bike when the show is on. You'll soon feel guilty if you watch television *without* cycling at the same time.

Some bicycling equipment, however, is so noisy that you must turn your television's sound up quite high. If you live in a house that won't be a serious problem, but in an apartment you might want to use an earphone or headset.

Many indoor cyclists listen to music while they ride, with good reason. Researchers at Ohio State University recently found that runners who work out to upbeat music described their exercise as "easier," even though it was at precisely the same workload. Their exercise was demonstrated to be less stressful physiologically when they combined it with music.

One indoor cyclist, who trains on rollers virtually every day, likes punk music because its heavy beat matches his fast cadence. Others enjoy disco music for the same reason. You also might want to try classical (the "1812 Overture" should get you moving), or country (but stick with upbeat tunes, not the "I'm blue because my honey left me for someone else" variety).

You might want to set up your indoor cycle near your stereo system so that you don't have to keep the speakers turned high in order to hear over the bike's noise. Or simply wear headphones or a tapeset (like Sony's Walkman) while you ride.

Once you're comfortable with your exercise program, you might develop your own tapes. Choose peppy, happy music (like the tunes used on aerobic dance records) and run the songs together for a continuous program. Choose tunes that you'll enjoy hearing over and over again. I especially like to cycle to the Pointer Sisters' energetic records.

You might even want to record tapes of certain lengths. Try a 20-minute tape, then a 30-minute one, maybe even a couple for 40. You could start each tape with 5 minutes of slower music (your warm-up), then a faster-paced 20- or 30-minute exercise segment, then a slower 5-minute cool-down. If you're really creative, stick in 1-minute intervals of very fast music (Rossini or "Footloose" comes to mind) for your interval work.

Special tapes designed for cyclists are being developed by Music in Motion. At the time of this writing, their bicycling tape was not yet completed, but their excellent, bouncy "Joggercise" tape is similar. Company president Raul Espinosa has carefully re-searched the types of music that keep you going and shorten your perception of how long you've been exercising. Steve Sokol plans to beat the World's Record of the most miles pedaled in 24 hours on an exercise bike while he listens to Music in Motion tapes.

Unfortunately, if you wear a heart beat monitor with head-phones, you'll be covered with wires. Don't suddenly jump off the bike to answer the phone—or you'll be the first indoor cyclist to trip over his own wires.

Cross-country record holder John Marino works out to mo-tivational and pep talks, some of which he tape-records himself. Others are prerecorded cassettes. Marino says these recordings have kept him going when all he wanted to do was crawl off the bike and go to bed.

If you try this, find tapes related to your exercise program ("I will get fit," "I will continue for another 15 minutes"), or try some that'll get you ready for further self-improvement (stop smoking, lose weight, learn assertiveness, and so on).

You also might want to sign up for fitness awards, whether in your local community or through a health club. YMCAs often post their members' progress in cycling and running programs. The President's Council on Physical Fitness also awards certificates to those who cover a certain number of miles by bicycle in a three-month period. Write to them for information.

Or take an occasional outdoor trip on a 10-speed bike. Cycling outdoors will add to your pleasure and demonstrate that you've developed a good base of fitness from your indoor program.

If the weather is nice, you might occasionally move your cycle out to the porch or backyard. Cycle on a sturdy surface, though, as most bikes are not easily adjusted to uneven ground or porches. However, don't leave your bike outdoors, since bad weather could ruin it.

John Marino's book also mentions friends of his who've developed interesting ways to combine indoor cycling with other activities. One, a lawyer, uses his reading stand to peruse court cases. Another, a professional photographer, sets up a slide projector with a remote control cord and a screen, then sorts his photos while exercising.

In addition, other unique ideas I've heard include: use your exercise time to dictate letters into a tape recorder for later transcription; talk on the phone (this works as long as you don't reach an anaerobic level, where you'll have trouble talking); or read homework assignments. Or, if you're Catholic, try saying the rosary while you ride. I understand that it's almost exactly 20 minutes long.

Take a hint from a study conducted by Gunnar Borg of Sweden's University of Stockholm. Borg found that monetary rewards produced an increase in maximal 45-second ergometer rides. As more money was paid for a ride, subjects were willing to increase the number of 45-second intervals they'd repeat.

You might, therefore, try self-bribery. If you ride for 20 minutes a day, for example, pay yourself $10 or $20, or perhaps a dollar a minute—money you can spend on whatever you like.

Finally, remember that plain old self-discipline is part of *any* exercise program. Naturally, you'll make indoor biking as intrinsically interesting as possible with these motivational tips. But there'll be days when you just don't *want* to ride. Recognize that those days will come, and get yourself up on that bike, no matter what.

9

How to Plan Your Fitness Program and Prevent Problems

PLANNING

Scheduling your exercise time and keeping to your schedule is the most important thing in your fitness program, especially at the beginning. You'll need about six weeks before you can feel you have safely established your routine so that it's become a habit. But if, right at the beginning, you don't set aside a certain time every day (or every other day) to ride your indoor bicycle, you won't do it. Too many other activities will intervene: the children have to be driven to their Scout meeting; you're starving after work and eat instead of exercising; a friend drops by and you end up chatting instead of cycling; or your spouse is late so you don't eat dinner until 8 o'clock, after which there's no time to ride your bike.

Sit down, right now, and examine your weekly schedule. When is the best time to ride your bike? I've found that if I don't ride my bike as soon as I get up, I just don't do it. At lunchtime I'm "too hungry." In the afternoon I'm "still digesting" my lunch. At dinner time I usually have a date or plans to visit friends, so I say, "I'll do it later." But I don't. I've now learned to predict my own behavior accurately enough that I *know* I must exercise first thing in the morning. I especially like that time because once I've "gotten my exercise out of the way," I can then plan the rest of the day without worrying whether I'll find time to ride my bike.

If, however, you have an early morning schedule that's so hectic that you'd have to get up at 4:00 A.M. to ride your bike, choose another time. Many people cycle indoors at lunch, whether they're at home watching the noon news, at work in their company's exercise room, or at a health club near their office. Or, if you get off work early, perhaps by 3:30 or 4 o'clock, that's probably the ideal time to ride your bike. It'll help you relax from work, and since it's too early for dinner, you won't have to worry about "digesting" after a meal.

If you arrive at home at 6 o'clock, fatigued from a strenuous day at the office, this might be the best time for you to hop on your bike and get oxygen circulating into your tired brain. A good exercise bout can reduce early-evening fatigue and lassitude and pep you up for your evening plans. Be sure not to eat dinner first, though.

Keep in mind that research studies show that exercising immediately *before* a meal cuts your appetite. Since dinner is the largest meal of the day for most people, you may lose weight, since you won't be as hungry.

If you're a night owl, you might want to wait two or three hours after dinner and then cycle. But try this schedule a few times before you adopt it, since some people find that exercising just before bed causes insomnia.

SLEEP

Be sure to get enough sleep, since beginning any kind of a fitness program puts a strain on your heart, muscles, tendons, and ligaments. Adequate rest is vital so that they recover completely from each day's exercise.

SHARING

If you will be sharing your exercise bike with your spouse and/or children, you'll need to work out a system to determine which miles belong to which family member. I'd suggest that each of you keep a log of your progress and write down all miles as they accumulate. You'll also want to mark your bike's seatpost (if it doesn't come numbered) so that you can put the seat precisely where it was the day before. You could use nail polish to mark the stem.

It's also possible that each member of the family might prefer a different saddle. Then, instead of taking off all the nuts and bolts every time you cycle, go back to your bike shop and purchase a seat post for each person. Then all you'll have to do is flip the quick-release lever to change the seat and the post.

If your family really gets involved, it might be fun to tack up a map of the United States with different-colored pushpins. It'll be obvious who's keeping up with their fitness program and who's not, since those who are will move across the map, while those who are not will stagnate. If your family has been idly mulling over the idea of taking a tour on 10-speed bikes, progress on the map will indicate who's ready to take on the outdoors and who isn't.

WOMEN'S SCHEDULES

Women should plan their programs a little differently from men, since some research indicates that women perform best aerobically during the first half of their menstrual cycle, and not so well as their period approaches. Since learning this, I've adjusted my fitness plan to cope with those monthly ebbs and flows of strength. Ever since, I've been able to maintain a high level of exercise throughout my monthly cycle and seldom feel sluggish when my period's due.

STARTING UP AGAIN

If you've caught a cold or the flu, or are recovering from another illness, doctors recommend that you not exercise until *at least* 24 hours after a fever has subsided. You may want to wait even longer, depending on how sick you've been. Your body simply *must* have time to recuperate before you can stress it again by bicycling, so force yourself to take a couple of days off.

When you come back to indoor cycling after a layoff, whether it was due to illness or a vacation, don't attempt to start at the same level at which you ended. If you haven't ridden your bike in a week, drop back a level. If it's been longer than that, drop back two levels. If, when you restart, you notice aches and pains that previously were not a problem, you might want to drop back another level. Don't worry about starting lower than where you left off—your stamina will return much more quickly than it did when you began your program.

NOISE

Some indoor bikes are considerably noisier than others. If you live in an apartment, place your exercise bike so that you won't wake your neighbors if you cycle at 7:00 A.M., or at midnight. Ideal locations are hallways near the front door, walk-in closets, bathrooms, kitchens, or virtually any room that's not above anybody else's bedroom or living room. If you've any doubt about how noisy your machine is, ask your neighbor. You may not have to ask, however—they'll probably tell you immediately.

PHYSICAL PROBLEMS

Minor Injuries

Many people start out too quickly in a fitness program and "burn out." They assume they're as fit as when they were 20, even though they're now 40. Or they expect to be able to keep up with a neighbor who's been cycling indoors for years.

The best way to avoid physical problems is to make sure that you keep a balance between training enough so you're challenged, yet not training so intensely that your underused muscles can't easily recuperate. See the schedules recommended in Chapter 5. Naturally, you want to set goals just slightly beyond your present reach. But remember that it's only a little beyond that stage to total exhaustion. And no one who's not a professional athlete should come anywhere near total exhaustion.

Exercise physiologists also suggest that if you plan to exercise almost every day, you should alternate hard days with easier ones. If, for example, you've started to intersperse some intervals with your endurance cycling, *don't* attempt to do intervals every day. You'll quickly burn out if you do. Experts recommend that you use intervals no more than once a week, at least until you are in top condition.

Typical minor injuries that you may encounter in an indoor cycling program include: saddle sores; aching sore muscles; and problems with your knees, back, neck, wrists, hands, and feet. Some simple cures are recommended here. However, if you continue to hurt, consult a doctor (preferably one familiar with sports medicine).

Although it's difficult to get seriously injured when riding indoor bicycling equipment, it can happen. I'll never forget the time one of my shoelaces worked itself loose without my noticing it, then suddenly tangled in the cranks. Without warning, my ankle was jerked to the side while the pedals continued to move. I quickly managed to stop the pedals and get myself untangled, but I briefly wondered how I would explain in the emergency room that I sprained my ankle on an indoor bicycle. Ever since then I've double-knotted my shoelaces before pedaling.

If you have a bike without a "freewheel" mechanism, be wary of pedals that continue to move when the flywheel moves.

People also have been injured by their saddles. Not long ago, the Consumer Product Safety Commission recalled hardware used to attach seats on 120,000 stationary bikes. Six people had been seriously injured when the metal seat post suddenly broke through the seat. Recalled were Scandi 462 bikes, sold by Sears as their model 2930.

A wobbling seat might be an indication that it's ready to come off. Be sure that *all* bolts are thoroughly tightened. If you're not too strong or not very handy with a wrench, get someone stronger to tighten your seat until it's immobile.

If you've purchased Schwinn's Air-Dyne, keep your eye on those moving handlebars when you start and stop the bike.

I've also heard horror stories of children and pets getting caught in wheel spokes before the indoor cyclist was aware they were nearby. This would especially be a problem if you ride a WLS or rollers. I'd suggest that you chain the dog, let out the cat, and put the baby in a playpen before you start to cycle.

Pain and Soreness

In addition to injuries, some cyclists just feel sore in various places. Although normally not a serious problem, soreness can destroy the best-planned indoor bicycling fitness program. Most soreness can be corrected by modifying your position on the bike or by changing the accessories you've been using.

SADDLE SORES

Saddle sores are probably the most common "injury" among indoor bike riders. See Chapter 4, where I suggest such preventive aids as special saddles, fluffy seat pads, and padded shorts.

Spenco has a chafing cream that reduces friction. It's made of silicone, formulated to leave a light barrier on your skin, and it's used by many professional cyclists—who often have serious problems with saddle sores.

In addition, be sure that your underwear is fresh and clean before you start pedaling. Many outdoor bicyclists also clean their crotch area with hydrogen peroxide before they cycle—an extra cleaning that ensures the entire area is free of bacteria that could cause irritation.

If you still have problems with saddle sores, you might also try various adjustments of your saddle's height and tilt. See Chapter 5 for a summary of these.

If you don't obtain relief, try a saddle like J.B.'s Easy Seat, where there's no friction between your legs since there's no *saddle* between your legs.

KNEE PAIN

Some indoor bicyclists have problems with their knees. Knee pain is usually due to riding rollers or a WLS in gears that are too low. Such gears force your knees to exert tremendous pressure to keep the pedals moving. You can have knee problems on a stationary bike or ergometer by pushing your legs to handle heavy workloads before they're ready to.

Still another way to bring on knee problems is to pedal too slowly. Research indicates that there's much less strain on your knees when you pedal at a cadence of 70 to 90 rpm than at lower cadences. Remember that you can do exactly the same amount of work at faster pedal speeds and lower tension, which definitely is easier on your knees.

Although cyclists are not nearly as prone to knee injury as are runners, there's still no reason to be injured if you can alter your workout to prevent it.

Other things to check if you're having knee pain are the size of your toe clips (too small ones are bad for your knees) and your shoes. Some people cannot cycle with normal jogging shoes, but have to have special cycling shoes to avoid knee pain. Remember, as Dr. I. Faria notes, when you're cycling on rattrap pedals "the pressure on the sole of the foot is in excess of 150 pounds per square inch."

BACK AND NECK PAIN

Pain in the back and neck also can occur if you're not comfortable on your bike. One ergometer I tested didn't have enough distance between the saddle and the handlebars. I always had the feeling of being "crunched up" in the saddle. I wanted to stretch out but had no room in which to do it.

If you're having any back pain, be sure to do sit-ups to strengthen your back. In addition, try adjusting your saddle slightly forward or back, and see if that helps.

WRIST AND HAND PAIN

Soreness or numbness of wrists or hands can also occur among cyclists. Although this kind of pain is more common if you ride your bike for more than an hour a day, you might have problems with any length of workout if your ulnar nerve is sensitive. This nerve branches when it reaches the wrist, and enters your hands in three different places. Resting your hands on your handlebars can compress it, resulting in weakness or tingling in your hands. If you have this problem, *don't ignore it*. Should this nerve deteriorate, it could result in permanent physical damage!

Fortunately, the solution is relatively easy. Purchase Spenco's or Grab-On's handlebar padding (*not* tape). I recommend both *very* highly. In addition to padding the bars, remember to move your hands around as you cycle. One of the major advantages of dropped handlebars is that there are so many places you can move your hands on those bars.

Should you still experience hand or wrist problems after you've padded your bars, consider wearing cycling gloves or Spenco's palm pads. Gloves and palm pads can be used as easily indoors as out, and they add yet another layer of padding between the bars and that sensitive ulnar nerve.

If you continue to have problems, I'd suggest you visit a doctor with a background in sports medicine. On this subject, Dr. Faria says: "If you do have to visit a doctor, don't forget to tell him that you are a cyclist and don't be bashful about your knowledge. . . . You could just be showing your doctor the first case that he or she has ever seen."

ACHING LEGS

If your legs feel sore for hours after you cycle, be sure to do *all* the stretching exercises before and after you ride (see Chapter 6). In addition, take a hot bath or shower after you've cooled down from cycling. A hot shower is terrifically soothing, and the heat helps relax tense muscles. I've tried cycling with and without stretching, and with and without a hot shower, and I've found that my muscles are more painful during the rest of the day if I forget to stretch or shower. Don't, however, immediately jump into a hot shower. Stretch, then walk around for a bit beforehand.

Miscellaneous Medical Problems

If you have hemorrhoids or herpes, you don't necessarily have to terminate your cycling program. Reread the section on saddle sores, and follow my suggestions.

Hemorrhoid sufferers might need to put some ointment on the affected area prior to cycling (after a thorough cleaning).

Research on herpes indicates that regular exercise may keep the disease from being as devastating as it is for those who don't follow a regular exercise program. Loose clothing, padding the affected area to prevent friction, and thorough cleansing may help. Your doctor can make the final recommendations on these problems.

WEATHER

The weather can also affect how you feel when you cycle indoors. Remember that your chances of exhaustion increase in climates where heat and humidity remain high throughout the summer. You can easily overexert yourself without realizing it. Although this is less likely to happen to indoor cyclists, it's still possible.

Be especially careful when the weather gets warmer overnight. This is when you're most vulnerable, since it takes a week or two for your body to acclimatize to increased heat and humidity. And research studies show that you don't become acclimated to hot weather unless you exercise in it.

You can drink as much as a quart of water before you cycle with no ill effect. In fact, in summer you should always drink that much before your workout. Some people even keep a water bottle on their indoor bike so that they can take a swig as they ride.

Temperature and humidity work together in much the same relationship as do cadence and workload: As one goes up, the other can stay the same and you'll feel more tired. And if both go up, you'll reach exhaustion more quickly.[1]

After the deadly summers of 1980 and 1983, the U.S. Weather Service issued a Heat Index chart. It tells you the temperature you actually "feel" when summer's heat is combined with sticky humidity (Figure 9–1).

Even though the temperature may stay the same, when the humidity increases, you feel hotter. In fact, you're in the chart's "alert" section at only 75°F—when the humidity hovers between 90 and 100 percent. The "caution" area begins at temperatures as low as 80°F, when combined with 95 percent humidity; "hazard" at 85°F and 95 percent humidity; and "danger" at only 90°F, when the humidity's 100 percent. A muggy St. Louis summer day of 90°F and 89 percent humidity will feel as hot as an 120°F Los Angeles scorcher.

The heat index chart is extremely important. Look it over carefully, and learn to use it. You might even photocopy it and tape it to your reading stand or nearby wall.

These readings are especially important if you have any type of heart disease, since the overload on your heart at higher humidity and temperatures can be severe. Learn the signs of heat exhaustion and heat stroke, and monitor yourself carefully. If in doubt, consult your doctor.

And don't *ever* wear one of those rubber or plastic exercise suits while cycling. It's extremely dangerous to sweat with no evaporation.

Your home or apartment doesn't need to be air-conditioned to follow a summer indoor bicycling program. Judicious arrangement of window and table fans will keep you comfortable in almost any kind of weather. I cycle without air conditioning, and there are only a very few days when I can't ride because my apartment

---

[1]G. Dimri, reporting in the *European Journal of Applied Physiology*, tested young Indian men already acclimatized to heat. They rode bicycle ergometers in conditions described as "comfortable," "hot humid," and "very hot humid." There was a significant increase in the oxygen cost of exercise as heat and humidity worsened, and they conducted more of the total exercise sessions in anaerobic rather than aerobic modes. Higher levels of lactic acid were also found as weather stress intensified, as was an increase in oxygen debt. The authors also found a significant reduction in maximum oxygen uptake under the "hot humid" and "very hot humid" conditions.

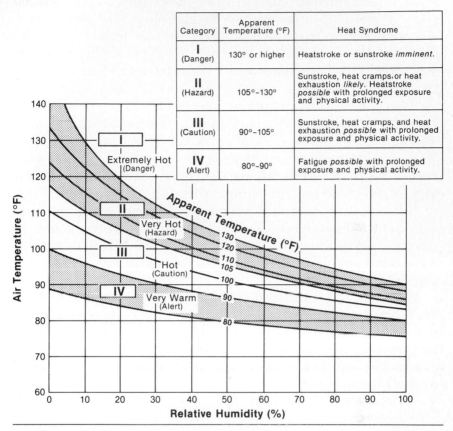

Category	Apparent Temperature (°F)	Heat Syndrome
I (Danger)	130° or higher	Heatstroke or sunstroke *imminent*.
II (Hazard)	105°–130°	Sunstroke, heat cramps, or heat exhaustion *likely*. Heatstroke *possible* with prolonged exposure and physical activity.
III (Caution)	90°–105°	Sunstroke, heat cramps, and heat exhaustion *possible* with prolonged exposure and physical activity.
IV (Alert)	80°–90°	Fatigue *possible* with prolonged exposure and physical activity.

Figure 9–1   Official U.S. National Weather Service Heat Index. (Reprinted with the permission of the U.S. Weather Service.)

is too hot. Of course, I ride early in the morning when the sun's low in the sky and my bedroom is still relatively cool.

Air conditioning, however, does make indoor exercise bearable during inclement summer weather. Some indoor cyclists place their bikes directly in front of the unit to obtain the full cooling benefit.

If you're going to cycle indoors without air conditioning, I suggest that you keep a thermometer next to your bike at all times, and always call the U.S. Weather Service's local recording to determine the humidity. Or you can purchase the temperature/humidity indicator discussed in Appendix A.

Naturally, you must make sure you don't get overheated when you cycle indoors in the winter. Some indoor bike riders open their windows, even on the coldest winter days, so as to ride comfortably. Others ride in the basement or garage, where it's cool year-round. My housemate and I turn down the heat when we go to sleep. In the morning, she's up and off early. I get up an hour later, then ride my indoor bike before I turn on the heat. If you live in an apartment where utilities are included, you might not be able to turn your heat up or down. In that case, either open a window or use a fan to keep yourself cool. Otherwise, you'll run the risk of becoming as overheated during winter cycling as you could on a hot summer day.

Unfortunately, there are still some apartments where you can't open the windows. Under those conditions, you may be able to run the air conditioner in the winter (I realize this sounds ridiculous, but do it anyway), or to set up a couple of fans to help cool you off.

Pollution alerts can affect your indoor cycling, especially if you don't use air conditioning. If you cycle in front of an open window that faces a polluted city street, follow the recommendations of the pollution alert exactly. If, however, you cycle where there's little traffic, just drop down a level in your program if the air is thick and heavy.

10

Indoor Bicycling, Physical Disabilities, and Aging

Many people in poor health, or people recuperating from illness or an operation, bicycle indoors. Indoor bicycling is also a very convenient means of staying fit for those who are deaf, blind, or have glaucoma, since for them other types of aerobic fitness programs may be dangerous or impossible without someone to guide them. The blind often cycle indoors accompanied by a metronome that keeps their cadence correct. The deaf prefer an indoor bike that has a light or timer which flashes when their workout is finished.

If you are recovering from an illness and need steady, predictable, and easily monitored exercise, you'll probably ride an exercise bike under the watchful eye of your physician or therapist. Numerous rehabilitation and physical therapy centers also employ indoor bicycles, since they provide the necessary precise measurements of exercise. The Veterans Administration Medical

Center in Northport, New York, for example, uses ergometers, as do many American hospitals.

Doctors, exercise physiologists, and rehabilitation therapists prescribe the exact levels of exercise to which their patients should adhere. Patients then keep exact exercise records, and progress to more intense levels very slowly.

Fitness levels of chronically institutionalized versus recently hospitalized patients were tested in a study reported by the *Journal of Gerontology*. The chronic patients had significantly lower heart rates and oxygen uptakes than did the newly admitted patients. After 12 weeks of training, significant improvements in fitness were noted in the chronic patients, who had exercised at only 50 percent of their maximum heart rate. The newly admitted men, however, showed little change at that workload. When the exercise intensity was increased to 60 percent, significant changes did occur for the new patients.

More and more doctors now recommend that heart patients or those with high blood pressure; arthritics; diabetics; asthmatics or people with allergies; those prone to backaches; and people with edema, multiple sclerosis, or even leukemia ride exercise bikes.

Patients recovering from operations (especially those for knees and hips, where it's difficult to find an exercise program that won't aggravate these joints), and people with varicose veins and ulcers also cycle indoors.

By the way, under no circumstances should anyone without a clean bill of health embark on any of the fitness programs in this book. If you have any physical problems, you *must* consult with your physician before embarking on an indoor bicycling fitness program. He or she will assist you in determining the proper combination of exercise, diet, medication, and (if unavoidable), surgery to best treat your problem.

A number of studies conclude that people who are more physically active have less heart disease than those who are less active. One researcher found five times as much total coronary heart disease among sedentary men when they were compared with other men who performed one or more hours of heavy work on the job every day. The actual severity of heart attacks also has been shown to be less among active men than among sedentary men.

Drs. William Haskell and Samuel Fox suggest that if a man moves from a "sedentary" category to an "intermediate" exercise level (which might mean a difference of only 100 to 200 calories per day in exercise), his risk of coronary disease drops significantly. They cite one study where men who performed up to 2 hours of "heavy physical work" daily had only 18 percent as much heart disease as did sedentary men.

Other studies have shown a similar correlation between strokes and physical activity. Men whose jobs require heavy physical work apparently have fewer strokes than do their sedentary coworkers.

Dr. William Castelli of the Framingham Heart Study in Massachusetts also recently observed the HDL (high-density lipoprotein) cholesterol levels of a group of cyclists. A high level of HDL cholesterol apparently helps keep artery walls clear, thus increasing blood flow to the heart and brain. He found that 25 miles of outdoor cycling per week produced a high amount of this "positive" HDL cholesterol in women.

A group of cardiac patients, the SCOR Cardiac Cyclists Club, takes regular bicycle outings in southern California. Randy Ice, a physical therapist and the club's president, says that the group uses *outdoor* bicycling as its major form of rehabilitation. "Most of these men have suffered an acute event, such as a heart attack, unstable angina, or bypass surgery," Ice said in a personal letter, "and have gone through a supervised monitored exercise rehabilitation program. Many of these patients started with stationary bicycles indoors, or ride their 10-speeds on American-made rollers manufactured by one of the members of our club."

"They are actually more physically fit than their middle-aged counterparts without heart disease," Ice says. He's also noticed "incredible" psychological changes in the group's members. "Every cyclist in the group has an improved sense of well-being and self-confidence. A strong sense of camaraderie and 'esprit de corps' exists among these men, and each helps the others overcome their own self doubts and anxieties," Ice says.

A study reported by the *Annals of Clinical Research* looked at changes from a fitness program designed for middle-aged men with borderline high blood pressure. Training lasted four months: The first two included supervised riding on a bicycle ergometer, the last two, unsupervised training. Both groups, the borderline and nonhypertensive controls, significantly increased their maximum oxygen consumption. They also both decreased their resting diastolic blood pressure. In fact, after training, the diastolic blood pressure in the borderline group didn't differ from that of normal men. The authors suggest that a fitness program is one mode of treatment for borderline hypertensive men.

Another study, this time at the University of Connecticut, found that regular exercise (which included calisthenics and pedaling a stationary bicycle) helped prevent osteoporosis (a bone disease that often strikes older women, and can result in rounded shoulders and loss of height).

A study on exercise and asthma, reported in the *Annals of Clinical Research*, suggests that exercise can be valuable for asthmatics, since it increases fitness levels and improves the asthmatic's self-image—and thus may reduce the number of attacks that are psychologically based.

One Swedish study mentioned by Dr. Samuel Fox in *The Bicycling Book* was conducted on people with edema. The researchers found that indoor bicycling can help reduce ankle swelling and improve circulation. Salesgirls who rode a stationary bike for 15 minutes each morning and afternoon had less swelling at day's end than did girls who didn't exercise.

A study reported in the *American Journal of Nursing* indicated that patients with Parkinson's disease can be helped by a comprehensive exercise program. Patients who rode an indoor bicycle showed reduced muscular rigidity and less depression after they commenced their exercise program.

Wheelchair-bound patients in Scandinavia have even learned to control their chairs better by training on a system of rollers that's similar to the rollers discussed in Chapter 3.

Doctors also frequently recommend indoor cycling for people who have been bedridden for long periods. There's even an indoor bicycle that you can ride in bed!

Research on the effects of bed rest reported by the National Aeronautics and Space Administration (NASA) found an increase in hypertension, reduced work capacity on a bicycle ergometer, and higher levels of calcium secretion. The first two effects were reduced if patients sat up or exercised and the third, by allowing them to stay upright for at least 3 hours a day.

Another study, also reported by NASA, found that five days of bed rest or 50 hours of sleep deprivation produced large decreases in heart and lung fitness. When subjects returned to a normal schedule of exercise, after two weeks they had only recovered about half the fitness level they'd lost.

Many senior citizens bicycle indoors, too. Residents of the Long Beach Senior Citizens Center ride Bodyguard ergometers, for example.

The president of the American Geriatric Society, Dr. Walter Bortz, recently examined more than 100 research studies, and concluded that the physical deterioration caused by aging is very similar to the deterioration that results from lack of exercise. In an article in the *Journal of the American Medical Association*, Bortz says that exercise helps prevent such deterioration, although, obviously, exercise can't prevent aging. In fact, he says: "Exercise is simple, cheap, and effective, which you can't say about many things in medicine. At least from a cardiac point of view, an activity program is a 40-year offset [to aging]. An active person of 70 is like an inactive person of 30."

If you know someone who's experienced one or more of the physical problems mentioned here and who despairs of ever becoming physically fit, show him this chapter. For safety's sake, however, be sure he consults with a doctor *before* beginning any of the suggested exercise programs in this book.

It's abundantly clear from current medical literature that physical disability (or increasing age) need not prevent anyone from achieving a high level of fitness via indoor bicycling, once they have a doctor's okay.

11

So You Want to Bicycle Outdoors

Although you didn't expect to get interested in cycling outdoors, you have. It happens to practically everyone who cycles indoors once their aerobic and muscular fitness has improved.

When you can easily put 20 or 30 miles on your indoor bike during a workout, and you've already cycled halfway across the United States, you begin to wonder just how well you'd do outdoors. How will those hills affect your speed? Will you learn to cope with those funny gears on your 10-speed bike? How will you react to the wind, to heat, and to humidity? Of course, you don't want to forget the greatest worry of all—crazy drivers!

You could continue your indoor bicycling program forever, without ever going outdoors or purchasing a 10-speed bike. But I'll bet once you've cycled in the "real world," too, you'll be hooked.

It's delightful to breeze along outdoors, watching houses, trees, joggers, scenic vistas, and other cyclists go by. I'll never forget the first time I cycled outdoors after I'd trained on my stationary bike for about six months. That was the easiest bicycling tour I'd ever taken. In fact, I actually got so interested in all the activity around me that I forgot I was bicycling! That had never happened to me before.

I hardly puffed as I surmounted hills. I breezed along flat streets and easily maintained 20 mph. I cycled almost 40 miles outdoors that day and didn't realize how far I'd gone until I sat down to calculate how many calories I'd burned.

What a contrast to a previous trip through the Maryland countryside of a few years ago! Then, since I hadn't followed an indoor exercise program, I was exhausted and sore after only 10 miles.

When you're in condition from indoor cycling, it's a joy and a delight to take a day-long trip outdoors on a Saturday or Sunday. Whether you plan your tour with topographic maps, or go on an outing sponsored by a local cycling club, you'll have a ball. And you might be surprised to discover that you're in far better condition than many cyclists you meet on the road.

Before you take off on a tour, however, here are a few facts that will help you enjoy your trip.

If you don't own a 10-speed bike, purchase one. Return to your trusted bike store, and see what they have in stock. I'd also recommend that you read two excellent books: John and Vera Krausz's *The Bicycling Book* and Eugene Sloane's *Complete Book of Bicycling* before you go. Sloane discusses the characteristics of a well-made touring bicycle in detail. Weight, for example, is of vital importance. You'll be propelling your bike, as well as your own weight, up hills. Lighter is better, but *don't* purchase a racing bike, the lightest of all. They aren't comfortable on long tours since they're very stiff.

You'll also want quality "components" on your bike: cranks, handlebars, pedals, seat, tire rims, and accessories. You'll want to pack at least one water bottle. If you plan to cycle lonely country roads in summer's heat, bring two or three bottles. Also buy a sturdy lock.

Use Sloane's book as a guide for your shopping.

Be sure to purchase the highest-quality helmet you can find. If you plan to ride without a helmet, I'd almost say you shouldn't ride outdoors at all. Accidents are common, and sometimes virtually unavoidable even if you're a defensive cyclist [I *always* assume drivers (1) don't see me and (2) are planning to make a sudden turn directly into my bike]. There will be times when you'll have to abandon your bike to survive.

An acquaintance of mine was cut off by a car that suddenly turned right while he was cycling through an intersection. He was thrown on his head. He wasn't wearing a helmet, since he "was only going to the Italian bakery for a loaf of bread." He's out of the hospital now, but the doctors are not sure how long it'll take for his headaches to go away, or for his sense of smell to return. Accidents can happen very quickly, especially if you're pedaling on city streets. Cycling without a helmet is foolhardy.

Your bike also should sport as many reflectors as you can fit on it. You may not plan to cycle at night (I don't recommend it), but when you're farther from home and more tired than you realized, you may end up cycling in twilight. Reflectors are essential safety equipment on an outdoor bike.

In addition, you'll want to carry U.S. Geological Survey topographic ("topo") maps in your bike bag. They're invaluable—especially when you've sailed down the biggest hill you've ever seen and aren't sure you can make it back up. Often when you pull out your topo map you'll find a nearby road that's virtually flat and leads back to where you started.

That happened to me on a solo trip one Fourth of July, when the humidity was 90 percent and the temperature 95°F. I was worried that I'd go into heat exhaustion if I tried to climb the massive hill I'd just coasted down. With the help of my topo map I managed to find another nearby route that was almost flat.

Also carry a jacket or sweatshirt in case a sudden storm blows up. Stick some identification in the pockets of your cycling shorts, too. My friend without the helmet who was in the accident wasn't carrying any ID. He was taken to a hospital, and only identified the next day when he was missing at work.

Bring a spare tire, and know how to change it. A tire pump is also helpful, unless you always cycle near gas stations. You'll probably want to add Grab-On or Spenco handlebar padding to your 10-speed bike, and if your saddle is new, pad that too. It's no fun to be 30 miles from home and have saddle sores so painful you can't cycle. Be prepared.

The cycling shoes, padded shorts, pulse monitor, bike computer, and gloves you've been using indoors can all go along outdoors. If you haven't purchased a bike computer, you probably will need a speedometer or odometer to keep track of the number of miles you've accumulated outdoors, as well as how fast you're cycling.

It's also fun to continue your training log as you cycle outdoors. Record your route, total miles, how long the trip took, temperature, humidity, and how you felt. Check your resting pulse the next day, to make sure that you didn't overdo it.

Before you go touring, you'll want to calculate your 10-speed's gear ratios. To find out how, refer back to the section "Aerobic Fitness Program: Rollers" in Chapter 5.

When cycling outdoors, try not to coast. Keep up the same cadence you use indoors, and change gears when your rpm is too slow or too fast.

Don't make the common mistake of pedaling long distances at low rpm in low gears. You'll tire very quickly and your knees will suffer.

Once you're on the road, there are a few variables you'll encounter that were irrelevant when you were cycling indoors.

First, hills. After months of training indoors, you'll buzz along flat stretches of road with ease. Hills, however, are another matter. If you've done some interval work with your aerobic program, however, your body should be somewhat prepared for hills.

Factors that affect your ability to climb hills include the weight of your bike and everything on it; *your* weight; the steepness of the hill; the pressure of your tires; and your level of fitness and amount of body fat. To climb hills more easily you can reduce the weight of your bike and its accessories to the bare minimum; lose weight (and fat); keep your tires pumped up to the recommended level; and work to improve your fitness level.

Drag, or air resistance, affects how fast you can travel comfortably. That's why you can't go 30 mph outdoors, as you perhaps can indoors. Headwinds and sidewinds also make a tremendous difference in your outdoor speed. Minimize the effect of the wind by riding low on the drops of your handlebars when appropriate. In addition, don't wear clothing that flaps in the wind. The next time you watch bike racers, note the slick, skintight clothing they're wearing. Research indicates that flapping clothing increases air resistance by as much as 30 percent.

Other variables that may disconcert you are traffic and dogs. With both, you can't be too cautious. Assume that all cars are going to hit you, and assume that all dogs bite. Then, when neither happens, you'll be pleasantly surprised.

Always cycle *with* traffic, not against it, and stay alert to traffic patterns. A rear-view mirror, mounted either on your handlebars or helmet, is invaluable for this.

As for dogs, many people carry cans of Halt and spray any dog that comes near them. For some reason bicycles fascinate unchained dogs, and you're bound to meet some of them if you cycle in the country.

If you want to try doing some intervals when you're cycling outdoors, time them from one telephone pole to the next, since that's safer than glancing at your watch. Most poles are spaced the same distance apart, so they provide good outdoor markers.

And don't forget to warm up, cool down, and stretch, just as you would when cycling indoors.

Also keep the temperature and humidity in mind. Remember that you're now out in the sun, which, on hot summer days, can quickly increase your internal temperature to a dangerous level. High outdoor temperatures, combined with high humidity, *can* be fatal.

Try to drink a water bottle full of water at least once an hour, every hour, when you're cycling in the heat. Be careful of suddenly overheating when you slow down or stop. The wind you generate while cycling keeps you cool when you're moving, but when you stop you feel the heat more intensely.

You should also be careful in cold weather. When you're riding a bike, the temperature doesn't have to be very cold for you to feel frozen. Cycling at 20 mph creates a wind-chill factor equivalent to a 20-mph wind. Cover your head and hands, and layer extra pairs of socks to keep your feet warm. And when it gets *really* cold, go back to cycling indoors.

If you want to work up gradually to longer outdoor tours, the American Youth Hostels (AYH) has a progressive chart that'll help you do so (Table 11–1).

Table 11–1   *American Youth Hostels Conditioning Plan for a 50-Mile Bike Tour*

1st day: 5 miles—Get acquainted with your bicycle. Rest every mile or two. Take about an hour.

4th day: 5 miles—Repeat the first day. Practice riding in a straight line.

6th day: 5 miles—Ride without stopping. Aim for half an hour.

7th day: 5 miles—Same as 6th day, but carry a 10-pound load.

10th day: 10 miles—Rest halfway only. Take 90 minutes.

12th day: 10 miles—No rest periods. Take one hour.

14th day: 25 miles—Rest 5 minutes every 5 miles. Take 3 hours.

17th day: 25 miles—Repeat 14th day but carry a 20-pound load.

20th day: 40 miles—Take your lunch. Rest every hour. Take 5 hours.

27th day: 50 miles—Take your lunch. Rest every hour. Take 5 hours.

28th day: 50 miles—Take all day. Carry full pack.

Source: Reprinted with permission from American Youth Hostels, Inc.

If you tour with the AYH or a local cycling group, don't feel obligated to discuss your indoor cycling program. I've found that people who only cycle outdoors sometimes take a condescending attitude toward those who train indoors. I can't explain their reasoning, but this attitude does exist. It's similar to talking to a runner who sets a 6-minute mile pace, when you're proud of jogging 10-minute miles; they simply don't understand your satisfaction and pride.

12

Bicycling (Indoors and Out) while Traveling and/or on Vacation

It may not be necessary to keep up an indoor cycling program while you travel or are on vacation, since recent research indicates it takes about 10 days before you lose the fitness level you've achieved.

If, however, you know you'll eat more than usual on your vacation or if you are taking a really long vacaton, you might want to stay at locations that offer stationary bikes or ergometers. The Sheraton Hotel system, for example, recently opened exercise rooms in many of its hotels. In Anchorage, Alaska; Zurich, Switzerland; Buenos Aires, Argentina; and Rotorua, New Zealand, Sheraton provides exercise rooms. If you want to be sure that they offer stationary bikes, contact a particular hotel directly. Sheraton's Press Information Coordinator didn't know which of their hotels had bikes and which did not.

Radisson Hotels were more informative. Their Lexington, Kentucky, hotel has a Schwinn XR-7 stationary bike, and their new Dallas, Texas, hotel has a stationary bike. Two of their resorts rent outdoor bikes. In addition, fourteen Radisson Hotels have special fitness areas, and they also offer low-calorie alternatives on every menu.

Hyatt Hotels provide "Aerobic Room Service" at some of their locations: You rent a stationary bicycle that's delivered to your room. Hyatt's "sports directory" lists all their fitness centers.

Marriott Hotels say that 80 percent of their locations offer exercise rooms. And even small hotels, such as St. Louis' English-style Cheshire Inn and Lodge, have exercise rooms with ergometers.

Even if your hotel doesn't have exercise bikes, you can probably walk or jog on a treadmill or outdoor trail, or at least work out in their weight room. If they don't have exercise bikes—why not suggest to them that they get some?

Perhaps you've considered a visit to a health spa and resort. Canyon Ranch in Tucson, Arizona, has two Monarks and a Schwinn Air-Dyne that are available at all times and which are incorporated into weight training classes. One of the Monarks boasts a pulse monitor. Canyon Ranch plans to add a Lifecycle bike to their exercise room sometime soon.

The Golden Door in Escondido, California, has a Dynavit Aerobitronic 20 and a Lifecycle. The Dynavit came with a pulse meter, and they attached one to the Lifecycle. Six stationary bikes are also available during supervised gym classes.

The Phoenix Spa in Houston, Texas, has two Schwinns (a Bio-Dyne and an XR-7) and a Monark. No modifications have been made to these bikes. All are located in their indoor track area, which also offers weight equipment, a tiny track, and an area for fitness classes. "Any bike that breaks down is replaced by a Schwinn Bio-Dyne bicycle," they say. "This is our preferred bike."

The Spa at Palm-Aire in Pompano Beach, Florida, has six Tunturi bikes and four Dynavits. They hope to order a Schwinn Air-Dyne in the future.

Cruise ships also have seen the virtues of indoor cycling. Cunard Line's *Queen Elizabeth 2* has Tunturis and Monarks aboard. (No modifications have been made to these bikes.) In addition, Cunard's *Princess* and *Countess* ships have Monark and Sears stationary bikes. (Again, no changes have been made to those bikes.)

If you're traveling by car and plan to stay at motels or hotels that don't provide stationary bikes, you might want to purchase a collapsible exercise bike. Monark's Spaar Rehab 858, a small stationary bike, weights 63 pounds and is fully collapsible. The seat post folds in half, as does the handlebar post, to produce a compact unit that could fit into the back of your car or station wagon.

If you "bring your own" indoor bike you'll join the ranks of professional athletes such as Kathy McMullen and Lynn Adams of the Ladies Professional Golf Association, who pack collapsible bikes as they travel on the LPGA tour.

I've never heard of anyone taking their stationary bike on a camping trip, but I suppose that's next.

Another idea, if you have a job where you travel to another city, then stay there for a month or so, is to rent a stationary bike from a bike shop for the time you're there. You might be able to work out a special two- or three-week rental price if they understand you're only in town for that long.

If you belong to a health club or YMCA in your hometown, check with them before you set out on your trip, since many offer free use of other health clubs throughout the United States. If so, you can write or call the ones in the city you'll be visiting, to see if they have exercise bikes available.

After you've followed the fitness program in this book for a while, you might consider a bicycling vacation—outdoors. It's easy to bring a 10-speed bike along on your trip, using a car carrier. Most major cities and recreational areas offer bike rentals, too. Just be sure to rent a bike that allows you to extend your legs completely. If possible, ask for a racing seat and touring handlebars. And a wrench, so you can raise the seat and handlebars.

Bring your kids along, too, either in child seats or on their own bikes. A tandem bike can even be adapted so your child can pedal in back with raised cranks that fit his or her shorter leg length.

National and international bike tours are available through a number of groups. One group you should contact is the League of American Wheelmen. This dynamic organization publishes a monthly magazine that includes a "cycling calendar" which lists dozens of tours and events throughout the United States. In a one-year span they listed more than 300 one-day tours, 80 week-end events, and almost 50 longer tours. In addition, members receive the LAW's directory, which is full of information on touring, as well as maps. It also lists 700 members who offer "hospitality homes," a kind of bed-and-breakfast system for cyclists. The directory also gives more than 500 bicycle touring groups throughout the country, and they'll help you start one if there aren't any nearby.

American Youth Hostels is another outstanding bicycling organization that plans tours in the United States and throughout the world. Virtually every weekend, members join local groups on trips from 5 to 200 miles, trips that fit your experience—no matter what it is. You receive a U.S. guidebook that shows all youth hostels (where the average age of guests often is 35), and, for a nominal cost, you can purchase hosteling guides to virtually every country in the world. The AYH also holds classes in beginning and advanced bicycle repair, which will help you prepare for a trip.

The International Bicycle Touring Society, headquartered in the United States, offers tours throughout this country and overseas. They'll teach you what to take, how to pack, everything you need to know about cycle touring in Europe, and suggest itineraries. Groups are only two to four people, and, according to their brochure: "You set your own pace and follow your own whims. Your only commitment is to be at the hotel in time for dinner." And, they say, "We have never lost anybody yet." Tours in 1983 included the California coast, the Poconos, the Finger Lakes in New York, the Smokies, and Florida, as well as New Zealand, England and Ireland, France, Switzerland, and Corsica. On some of the IBTS tours, such as a recent one to Greece, the average age of the cyclists was as high as 62!

A new touring group, affiliated with the IBTS, was recently created. Known as the Bicycle Adventure Club, it now has fifty members. They plan tours of a more adventurous nature than those of the IBTS.

Another organization, Bicycle Detours, schedules "discovery vacations" on all-terrain mountain bicycles. These bikes are 15-speed models with wide tires, so you follow rugged mountain paths. Frank and Sarah Lister say: "You don't have to be an experienced cyclist to enjoy yourself." Many of their tours include back-country sites of archaeological interest in the southwestern United States.

Another group that can be of tremendous assistance in planning U.S. tours is Bikecentennial. They can tell you about bicycle routes, such as the 4450-mile TransAmerica Bicycle Trail, the Great Parks Bicycle Route, The Great River Cycle Route along the Mississippi, and 300-mile loop routes in Oregon, Kentucky, and Virginia. Bikecentennial plans summer group tours of eight to ten cyclists, ranging in duration from 21 to 90 days. Members also receive a *Cyclists' Yellow Pages*, a guidebook that helps you plan your own bike tours.

If you're yearning for the British Isles, contact England's Cyclists' Touring Club. Their delightful magazine, *Cycletouring*, covers all aspects of touring in the United Kingdom, and has occasional articles about European touring. The classified ads are fascinating, and you could plan your British tour around the bed-and-breakfast homes listed therein. This magazine also has a terrific selection of books, maps, and a library of routes throughout Europe recommended by members, to add to the pleasure of your British tour. They'll even help you plan "Fixed Center Tours," where you take daily cycle tours in the area near your hotel. The CTC sponsors organized tours every year that usually consist of twelve to sixteen people. Information on upcoming summer's tours is published in their December issue. They've even organized some thematic tours, including "Castles of Wales" and "A Fortress Tour of Northumberland and Scotland."

Bike Tour France, a group headquartered in the United States, leads tours of France in spring, summer, and fall. Director Jerry Simpson lived in France for a few years and is intimately familiar with French language and culture. One of his most exciting tours is a "Wine Country Tour," which includes a new bike, accommodations for fifteen nights in some of the most beautiful chateaux in the country, fourteen dinners and nine lunches, boat transfers, numerous wine tastings, and "lots of extras."

Or perhaps cycling in Australia or New Zealand appeals to you. Active cycling organizations exist in both countries. You'll want to subscribe to *Freewheeling* magazine, which features numerous interesting articles on cycle tours in Australia (a country that's as large as the United States). The magazine's catalog offers fascinating books about bike tours to such places as Melbourne, Victoria, New Zealand, and the Blue Mountains. You can even purchase *The Kid's Book of Bicycles in Australia* and get your children enthusiastic about touring the country.

If you've always had a yen to visit South Africa, the Pedal Power Foundation of southern Africa will help you plan a tour. Their magazine, *Velocipede*, is published by volunteers, written for the noncompetitive cyclist, and covers touring extensively.

Should you be traveling and simply can't work in any indoor or outdoor bicycling, you might want to try other aerobic fitness activities. Swim laps at your motel's pool, or go jogging on nearby paths. Hike in the woods, or cross-country ski when the weather's right.

But go *slowly* with alternate fitness programs since running, swimming, hiking, and cross-country skiing stress different muscles than you've been using on your indoor bike. Start slowly, and give your tendons and ligaments a chance to adapt. Remember that your goal is to stay fit, *not* to pull a muscle that will spoil your trip.

Have a healthy, fit vacation.

Appendixes

APPENDIX A: OTHER USEFUL ACCESSORIES

Bicycling Shoes

Some bicycling shoes look funny. They're not made to be walked in, although there now are some models in which you can take a short hike. Some cycling shoes are made to be worn with "cleats," metal attachments that fit on your shoes and match up with the pedals. Cleats aren't necessary for indoor cycling, since you use toe clips and straps. But if you plan to use cleats on your 10-speed bike, it makes sense to purchase shoes to fit them. Cycling shoes run about $30. Cannondale makes a nice pair.

Spenco makes a sturdy pair of "orthotics" that cyclists can put into their sneakers or running shoes to make them stiff enough to cope with metal pedals. And you won't have to buy a special pair of cycling shoes if you use these excellent $15 insoles. I highly recommend them, and use them almost every day.

Another insert, the Power Flex Bicycle Insert, is made with layers of plastic, stainless steel, and foam that form a stiff base. It's $13 and available from the Sunflower Group.

Gloves

I've found that with padding on my handlebars I'm perfectly comfortable, with no wrist or hand pain. However, your hands and wrists might be more sensitive than mine. In that case, I'd recommend cycling gloves designed to prevent hand fatigue.

Spenco, those masters of innovation, now have both gloves and "palm pads" for cyclists. Both are made of the same soft, spongy material that's used in their terrific saddle pads. The gloves have a leather upper, while the small palm pads are for people who don't want to wear gloves or who need extra padding when wearing gloves made by other manufacturers. The cost is about $6.

Other gloves have leather palms and cotton on a mesh area over the back of your hands. Many have a Velcro strap, and some have padding that extends up the thumb. Bike Nashbar makes a nice pair at $6, and another, even thicker, for $14.

Heartbeat Monitors

If you don't want to take your pulse by hand, heartbeat monitors can record fluctuations in your heart rate. Some display your previous heart rate electronically, while others buzz if you exceed a preprogrammed maximum pulse.

Heartbeat monitors come in a number of designs. One attaches to the handlebars, and you slip your fingertip into a housing to obtain a reading. Another attaches to your chest, and your pulse is constantly displayed with a digital readout. Others hook to your earlobe or have sensors that pick up your pulse while your hands rest on the handlebars. There's even a "wristwatch" gadget that digitally reads out your pulse as you exercise.

A heartbeat monitor could be helpful if your doctor recommends that you follow a precisely regulated cycling program. All you have to do is watch the monitor to see if you're overexercising. If you're overdoing, slow down. Or if you're not working hard enough to raise your pulse to the recommended level, your monitor will indicate that.

Monitors are useful if you're one of those people who just can't find your pulse, no matter how hard you try. If, however, you've had trouble locating your pulse, try again while you're exercising before you buy a heartbeat monitor. Your heart rate is much more difficult to locate when you're resting than when you're exercising.

Consumer Reports tested monitors twice, in January 1980 and again in July 1981. They suggest that you save your money and count your pulse with a wristwatch instead. Dr. Ed Burke agrees, stating that a monitor must be a chest unit, and expensive, to be accurate.

Pulse monitors were rated by *Bicycling* magazine in April 1982, and they found that monitors could vary by as much as 60 beats when their testers moved around.

Some monitors don't give accurate readings if you're moving (as you would be, if only slightly, on an exercise bike), or if your hands are dirty or dry. Many monitors take 10 to 20 seconds to register an accurate heart rate, long enough for you to count your pulse manually.

The Exersentry Heart Rate Monitor has been praised by the U.S. Nordic Ski Team, who describe it as "a fine product indeed," and by Dr. Thomas Dickson at the Cycling and Fitness Center in Emmaus, Pennsylvania. This $170 heartbeat monitor, which is worn strapped to your chest, offers an alarm that sounds when you are above your maximum or below your minimum recommended levels (see Chapter 5).

The price of heartbeat monitors may convince you of the virtues of taking your pulse by hand, as I do.

Bicycle Computers

Computers abound for cyclists, just as they do for everyone else. Virtually all bicycle computers on the market attach to the front (and sometimes rear) wheel of a 10-speed bicycle. Therefore, if you've purchased an exercise bike or ergometer, you won't be able to use a computer. Nevertheless, if you have a WLS or rollers, you might be interested in a computer—or you might want one for your 10-speed bike. It's quite possible that computers will replace speedometers and odometers sometime soon.

The three computers mentioned here all measure your rpm rate, a useful feature.

Attivo's Push computer is the smallest of the bunch, and a kit is available to convert it for use on a WLS. The Push weighs only 3.5 ounces, and measures $3\frac{1}{2}$ inches by 2 inches, a size that fits nicely on your handlebars without taking up too much space. Using this computer, you'll know your speed (from 0 to 70 mph), cadence up to 135 rpm, the cumulative trip and total distances, and the time of day. It also acts as a stopwatch. Extended battery life is a nice feature, and you don't lose cumulative data when you change your battery. It's quick-release, so you don't have to leave it on your 10-speed bike if you're outdoors. I also like the ridges on each button, so that you know you're pressing the correct one. The Push sells for $60.

The Pacer 2000 keeps you apprised of elapsed time, distance traveled, rpm speed, average speed, and heart rate, and acts as a stopwatch. To obtain a heart rate readout, you'll strap an optional belt around your chest. John Marino, holder of numerous cross-country cycling records, says: "The most valuable tool on my record ride was the computerized feedback I got from my Pacer 2000." It sells for $99, plus $60 for the heart belt kit.

Another computer, the Coach, rates your fitness level (via maximum oxygen uptake), shows pulse, counts the calories you've burned, beeps when you're in your aerobic range or when you're exercising at too high a pulse rate, shows elapsed time and distance, and your speed. You'll need to purchase a bicycle adapter for this computer. It's expensive: $250 plus $35 for the bike adapter.

Videogame Joystick

The latest accessory for your stationary bike or ergometer is an Aerobics Joystick. This "exercycle interface," as the manufacturers call it, works on Schwinn and other stationary bikes and connects to an Atari 2600, 400/800/1200, or Sears Telegame. The cost is about $40.

"In Activision's Enduro game," they say, "the faster you pedal, the faster your car will go. It will seem as if you are there inside the screen, pedaling through a 24-hour endurance race, steering past obstacles and other cars. . . . After a while, you won't know that you are exercising, you will only know that you're having a great time."

You also can "play" other road-racing and "shoot-'em-up" games such as "Missile Command" and "Defender" with the joystick. In fact, *American Health* magazine says: "Test subjects have had so much fun sweating over the Aerobics Joystick that they're dusting off their nearly forgotten exercycles."

If you plan to work out with the joystick, however, be sure to keep an eye on your pulse, since it would be easy to get so involved that you'd exceed 85 percent of your maximum pulse. Be careful.

Tire Pump

If you're using a WLS with rollers, or riding rollers, you'll need to keep your bicycle tires extremely hard. After a couple of trips to a gas station to pump up my tires (since my small Zefal pump simply couldn't cope), I purchased Schwinn's foot pump with a reservoir for $28. With this new pump design, extra air that normally whooshes from your tires doesn't; instead, it whooshes into the *reservoir*, and your tires don't deflate when you remove the pump.

I can't recommend this pump too highly. It's almost a necessity when you're riding rollers, since even slightly flat tires produce a terrible ride.

Temperature and Humidity Indicator

If you really get involved with indoor cycling, you might want to purchase a Deluxe Hygrometer and Temperature Indicator. Quill Corporation sells these in their office supplies catalog. Although designed for computer rooms where machines are highly sensitive to heat and humidity, they function just as well as a supplement to an indoor bicycling program. (See Chapter 9 for a detailed discussion of how temperature and humidity can affect your fitness program.)

This indicator is especially nice if your home doesn't have air conditioning. The thermometer only reads up to 100°F, however, and last summer in St. Louis we exceeded 100°F for almost twenty days! Plan to spend about $80 for this hygrometer—but that sure beats trying to get through to the continually busy U.S. Weather Service lines.

APPENDIX B: RELEVANT BOOKS

The Aerobics Program for Total Well-Being by Kenneth H. Cooper, M. Evans and Company, Inc., New York, 1982. An excellent book on the subject of aerobics, which explains his "point system" in detail. $15.95 hardcover.

The All New Complete Book of Bicycling by Eugene A. Sloane, Simon and Schuster, New York, 1981. This is "the" book on bicycling and bike repair. Read this before you choose a 10-speed bike, and then read it again when you're planning a tour or need to repair your bike. It's comprehensive and covers the subject in exhausting detail. $19.95 hardcover.

Anybody's Bike Book: An Original Manual of Bicycle Repairs by Tom Cuthbertson, Ten Speed Press, Berkeley, Calif., 1971. A good basic bike-repair book for your 10-speed bike which features simple explanations. $4.95 paperback.

Beyond Diet . . . Exercise Your Way to Fitness and Heart Health by Mazola Corn Oil, Dept. RF-C, Box 307, Coventry, CT 06238. Ask for a copy of this excellent pamphlet. Free.

The Bicycling Book: Transportation, Recreation, Sport by John and Vera van der Reis Krausz, eds., Doubleday & Company, Inc., New York, 1982. An outstanding book that covers virtually every aspect of bicycling, indoors and out, although mostly out. You'll learn the rules of the road, how to tour, basics of bike riding, how to train and stay fit, how to deal with injuries, and so on. Highly recommended—a "don't miss." $11.95 paperback.

Bicycling Science by Frank Rowland Whitt and David Gordon Wilson, The MIT Press, Cambridge, Mass., 1982. Although this book can get quite technical, its discussion of human power generation, heat transfer, wind resistance, braking, balancing, and unusual bikes is worth the price. $9.95 paperback.

Cycling Physiology for the Serious Cyclist by Irvin E. Faria, Charles C Thomas Publisher, Springfield, Ill., 1978. A comprehensive study of human physiology and its relation to bicycling that's comprehensible to the average reader. $13.95 hardcover.

A Diet for Living by Jean Mayer, David McKay Company, Inc., New York, 1975. A terrific general guide to healthy eating by the author of the excellent book *Overweight*. Dr. Mayer is a man you can trust to give you accurate facts, without hype. $8.95 hardcover.

The Fitness Fact Book: A Complete Guide to Diet, Exercise, and Sport by Theodore Berland, The New American Library, Inc., New York, 1980. An excellent discussion of all aspects of exercise and fitness, with ratings of various exercise regimens and of equipment. A terrific companion to his fine book *Rating the Diets*. $2.25 paperback.

Get Fit with Bicycling by the editors of *Bicycling* magazine, Rodale Press, Emmaus, Pa., 1979. A collection of articles and questions and answers from the magazine, all related to nutrition and fitness. $3.95 paperback.

Inside the Cyclist: Physiology for the Two-Wheeled Athlete by the editors of *Velo-news*, *Velo-news*, Brattleboro, Vt., 1982. A compendium of articles that appeared in previous issues of the magazine, on diet, training, injuries, and general cycling physiology. Easy to read and informative, it includes some outstanding articles by Dr. Ed Burke. $7.95 paperback.

International Cycling Guide by Nicholas Crane, ed., The Tantivy Press, 136–148 Tooley Street, London SE1 2TT, England, or A. S. Barnes & Company, Inc., San Diego, Calif. Also distributed by *Bicycling* magazine. An annual book that tells you about new bikes, racing, touring, and trends, and has incredible details on groups, museums, mail-order firms, and magazines throughout the world. $9.95 paperback.

John Marino's Bicycling Book by John Marino, Jeremy P. Tarcher, Inc., Los Angeles, 1981. $6.95 paperback.

North American Bicycle Atlas by American Youth Hostels, 3rd ed., Delaplane, Va., 1973. This book is full of tours, trips, and treks throughout the United States and abroad. No matter where you plan to vacation, you'll find a tour in here. $2.50 paperback.

Nutrition, Weight Control, and Exercise by Frank I. Katch and William D. McArdle, Lea & Febiger, Philadelphia, 1983. A fine book to read if you're concerned about keeping your weight under control. Excellent discussion of body fat and how to calculate it, with extremely detailed tables. $18.50 paperback.

Overweight: Causes, Cost, and Control by Jean Mayer, Prentice-Hall, Inc., Englewood Cliffs, N.J., 1968. The best book on the subject so far. Dr. Mayer is internationally known for the quality of his research on the subject of weight loss. Out of print; check your library.

Pedal Power by James C. McCullagh, Rodale Press, Emmaus, Pa. 1977. A fascinating look at the incredible variety of uses to which a stationary bike can be put, mostly generating energy in underdeveloped countries. Out of print; check your library.

The Physiology and Biomechanics of Cycling by Irvin E. Faria and Peter R. Cavanagh, John Wiley & Sons, Inc., New York, 1978. An excellent book, written so that most average readers can understand it, detailing the physiology of cycling. $15.95 hardcover.

Rating the Diets by Theodore Berland, *Consumer Guide* Publications, 3841 West Oakton Street, Skokie, IL 60076. Another annual book that rates all currently popular weight-loss diets from the most sensible to the most bizarre, with pros and cons of each. Berland is the only author providing this important rating service to the public. This book is highly recommended. $3.95 paperback.

Rating the Exercises by Charles T. Kuntzelman, Penguin Books, New York, 1980. The author rates all exercise programs for *Consumer Guide* magazine in this useful book. $3.95 paperback.

The Wilmore Fitness Program: A Personalized Guide to Total Fitness and Health by Jack H. Wilmore, Simon and Schuster, New York, 1981. Full of good recommendations on how to incorporate exercise, particularly calisthenics, into your daily life. $8.95 paperback.

APPENDIX C: BICYCLING PUBLICATIONS

The Bicycle Paper
P.O. Box 842, Seattle, WA 98111. The only newspaper for cyclists in the northwestern United States.

Bicycle Sport
Wizard Publications, 3162 Kashiwa Street, Torrance, CA 90505. 213-539-9213. One of the best of the new cycling magazines, it includes fascinating interviews, recommended tours, health information, and lots more.

Bicycling
Rodale Press, Emmaus, PA 18049. The thick, glossy magazine of cycling.

Cycling
Surrey House, 1 Throwley Way, Sutton, Surrey SM1 4QQ, England. Bicycling racing magazine from England.

Cyclist
P.O. Box 993, Farmingdale, NY 11737. 800-645-9559 or 800-732-9119 in New York. A new magazine which covers touring, racing, equipment, and health.

Freewheeling
Freewheeling Australia Publications, P.O. Box K 26, Haymarket, New South Wales 2000, Australia. This magazine is published bimonthly, and is chock full of information on cycle touring in Australia and New Zea-

land. Be sure to get a copy of their mail-order catalog. Their touring service is the only information service available on touring conditions in Australia, and they'll send packets with maps, articles, and brochures on particular areas.

Velo-news

Box 1257, Brattleboro, VT 05301. 802-254-2305. An outstanding publication, with extensive covering of training and racing.

Velo Press

c/o Canadian Cycling Association, 333 River Road, Vanier, ON, K1L 8B9, Canada. 613-746-5753. Touring and racing in French and English. Order a copy of *Cycle Canada a Velo*, a guide to cycling trips in that country.

Winning Bicycle Racing Illustrated

1127 Hamilton Street, Allentown, PA 18102. 215-821-6864. They say that they are the "single best-selling bicycle racing publication, of any language, in the world." Founded in 1983.

APPENDIX D: BICYCLING AND FITNESS ORGANIZATIONS

American Youth Hostels

1332 I Street, NW, No. 800, Washington, DC 20005. 202-783-6161. An excellent group that you don't have to be a "youth" to join. Active local councils promote bicycling, hiking, and canoeing, and offer tours of the United States and overseas. Leadership training classes are available, as are guidebooks. Membership is $20, families $30.

Australian Amateur Cycling Federation

c/o Ron L. O'Donnell, 20 Paterson Crescent, Morphettville, South Australia 5043, Australia. Phone 08-295-6178. The governing body of amateur cycling in Australia.

Bicycle Adventure Club

515 Vista Flora, Newport Beach, CA 92660. New branch of the International Bicycle Touring Society that sponsors tours of a more "adventurous" nature.

Bicycle Detours

P.O. Box 44078, Tucson, AZ 85733. 602-326-1624. You can tour Arizona, New Mexico, Utah, Colorado, even Mexico on all-terrain mountain bikes.

Bike Tour France

P.O. Box 32814, Charlotte, NC 28232. 704-527-0955. Excellent tours of France offered spring, summer, and fall.

Bikecentennial

P.O. Box 8308, Missoula, MT 59807. 406-721-1776. Maps and a detailed catalog of books on cycling are available.

Cycletouring

c/o Cyclists Touring Club, Cotterell House, 69 Meadrow, Goldalming, Surrey GU7 3HS, England. This is the magazine of the Cyclists Touring Club of England, which sponsors tours and provides information about tours in the United Kingdom and on the Continent. Highly recommended. Membership is £10.

International Bicycle Touring Society

2115 Paseo Dorado, La Jolla, CA 92037. 714-291-1258 or 714-291-2108. Membership is $10 (single or couple). They organize trips throughout the United States and overseas, in small-group format.

League of American Wheelmen

P.O. Box 988, Baltimore, MD 21203. 301-727-2022. They plan numerous tours throughout the United States and have local groups in most large cities. Membership is $18; family $24.

The Pedal Power Foundation of Southern Africa

35 Forth Road, Rondebosch 7700, South Africa. They publish a magazine called *Velocipede* on a quarterly basis, for noncompetitive cyclists, which covers touring, bicycle facilities, and local news. A good source of information if you plan to visit that country.

President's Council on Physical Fitness and Sports

450 Fifth Street, NW, No. 7103, Washington, DC 20001. 202-272-3430. Ask about their awards for bicycling.

SCOR Cardiac Cyclists Club, Inc.
c/o Randolph Ice, R.P.T., Presbyterian Inter-Community Hospital, 12401 East Washington Boulevard, Whittier, CA 90602. 213-698-0811, ext. 2635.

United States Cycling Federation
1750 East Boulder Street, Colorado Springs, CO 80909. 303-632-5551. They govern both amateur and professional cycling in the United States and are strongly involved in all aspects of racing.

APPENDIX E: MANUFACTURERS: ACCESSORIES AND EQUIPMENT

Aerobics Joystick
Suncom, Inc., 650 East Anthony Tr., Northbrook, IL 60062.

Biocycle/Engineering Dynamics Corporation
120 Stedman Street, Lowell, MA 01851. 617-458-1456.

Bodyguard/J. Oglaend, Inc.
40 Radio Circle, Mt. Kisco, NY 10549. 914-666-2272, 800-828-1186.

Cannondale Corporation
9 Brookside Place, Georgetown, CT 06829. 203-838-4488.

Coach
BioTechnology, Inc., 6924 NW 46th Street, Miami, FL 33166. 800-327-1033 or 305-592-6069.

Easyseat
JB Two Corporation, P.O. Box 6025, St. Paul, MN 55118. 612-699-0786.

Exersentry Heart Rate Monitor
Respironics, Inc., 650 Seco Road, Monroeville, PA 15146. 414-373-8114.

Grab-On
100 North Avery, Walla Walla, WA 99362. 509-529-9800.

Kreitler Rollers
5102 Bannister Road, Kansas City, MO 64137. 816-765-0635.

Lifecycle, Inc.
10 Thomas Road, Irvine, CA 92714. 714-859-1011.

Monark/Universal Fitness
20 Terminal Drive South, Plainview, Long Island, NY 11803. 516-349-8600.

MTD Rollers (also see Bike Nashbar catalog)
Modern Line Products Co., P.O. Box 110, Indianola, MS 38751.

Music in Motion
P.O. Box 2688, Alameda, CA 94501. 415-430-0618.

Novel Products, Inc. (Fat-O-Meter Skinfold Caliper and Tape Measure)
80 Fairbanks Street, Addison, IL 60101. 800-323-5143; in Illinois 312-628-1787.

Pacer 2000
Veltec, P.O. Box 1156, Fort Collins, CO 80522. 303-221-3035.

Perceptronics LaserTour
6271 Variel Avenue, Woodland Hills, CA 91367. 213-884-7470.

Power Flex Bicycle Insert
The Sunflower Group, Inc., 804 Massachusetts Street, Lawrence, KS 66044.

The Push
Attivo Corp., P.O. Box 852, 320 Main Street, Longmont, CO 80501. 303-772-8598.

Quill Corporation
100 South Schelter Road, Lincolnshire, IL 60069. 312-634-4800. Office supply catalog (source of the hygrometer, which shows humidity and temperature).

Racer-Mate
3016 NE Blakely Street, Seattle, WA 98105. 206-524-7392.

Schwinn/Excelsior Fitness Equipment Co.
613 Academy Drive, Northbrook, IL 60062. 312-291-9100.

Spenco Medical Corp.
P.O. Box 8113, Waco, TX 76714. 800-433-3334; in Texas 817-772-6000.
Ask about local dealers who carry their gloves, palm pads, saddle pad,
handlebar padding, and inserts.

TurboTrainer
SkidLid Specialties, Inc., 1560 California Street, San Diego, CA 92101.
714-234-4244.

APPENDIX F: MAIL ORDER CATALOGS

The Bicycle Exchange
3 Bow Street, Cambridge, MA 02138. 617-864-1300.

Bike Nashbar (formerly Bike Warehouse)
215 Main Street, New Middletown, OH 44442. 800-345-BIKE to place
an order, or 216-542-3671. One of the best mail-order firms, with a
comprehensive catalog and very prompt, reliable service. Highly recommended.

R. J. Chicken & Sons Ltd.
Bisley Works, Landpark Lane, Kensworth, Dunstable, Bedfordshire LU6
2PP, England. A glossy catalog from England.

Endurance Sports
2206 South 2000 West, Salt Lake City, UT 84119. 800-874-6740 or 801-
972-8740.

The Handbook of Cycl-ology
2745 Hennepin Avenue South, Minneapolis, MN 55408. 612-872-7600.
$3 for a huge catalog.

Lickton's Cycle City
310 Lake Street, Oak Park, IL 60302. 800-323-4083 or 312-383-2130.

Money Order Mail Order (M.O.M.O.)

P.O. Box 181, Glencoe, IL 60022.

Palo Alto Bicycles

P.O. Box 1276. Palo Alto, CA 94302. 800-227-8900 or 415-328-0128.

Pedal Pushers

1130 Rogero Road, Jacksonville, FL 32211. 800-874-1736; in Florida 800-342-7320.

Performance Bicycle Shop

1126 Sourwood Drive, P.O. Box 2741. Chapel Hill, NC 27514. Accessories, rollers, and wind-load simulators in this catalog.

Touring Cyclist Shop

2639 Spruce Street, P.O. Box 4009, Boulder, CO 80306. 303-449-4067.

Two Wheeler Dealer

4406 Wrightsville Avenue, Wilmington, NC 28403. 800-334-1612 or 919-799-6444.

Wandering Wheels Cyclery

5211 North 38th Street, P.O. Box 09164, Milwaukee, WI 53209. 414-466-0358.

Index

Catalog

If you are interested in a list of fine Paperback
books, covering a wide range of subjects
and interests, send your name and address,
requesting your free catalog, to:

McGraw-Hill Paperbacks
1221 Avenue of Americas
New York, N.Y. 10020